A Life Changing Companion

Journey Guide

for Caregiver Support Groups
or Individual Study

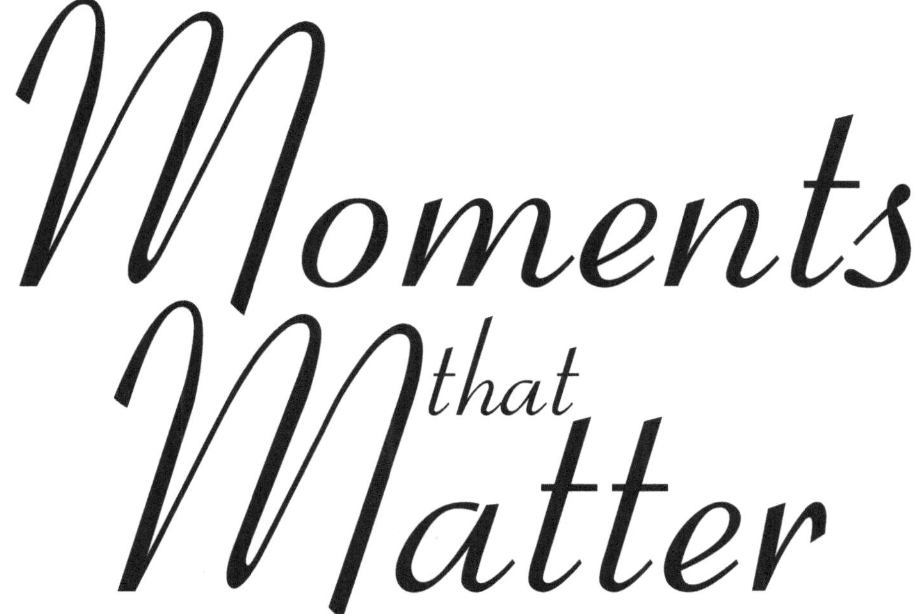

Moments that Matter

KAREN COCHRAN BEAULIEU

ISBN 979-8-88644-257-1 (Paperback)
ISBN 979-8-88644-258-8 (Digital)

Covenant Books
11661 Hwy 707
Murrells Inlet, SC 29576
www.covenantbooks.com

Dedicated to the most vibrant of all hummingbirds,

Betty Moore Cochran

She fluttered her wings from October 31,1920-August 5th, 2022

A mother so loved…a daughter so blessed

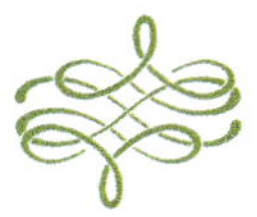

Sweet Melody

A vibrant little hummingbird
the flutter of her wings are heard
she gathers scents of yesteryear
the changing of her life unclear
unsure about her paths of flight
her journeys are a constant fight
confused about so many things
or could it be a broken wing?

I know this wing will never heal
I wonder how her heart must feel
a poet searching for a rhyme
trapped in a fog within her mind
everything seems quite absurd
this broken little hummingbird

If only someday I could be
inside her mixed reality
perhaps I would unravel why
she wonders why the monarchs fly
or why the yellow songbird sings
she just forgets so many things

I'd know I'd find her mind carefree
sweet nectar is her melody
she lives her life quite happily
entwined with fragrant memories

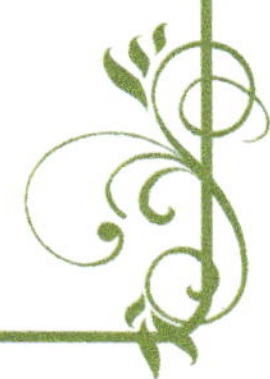

kcb

In Loving Memory

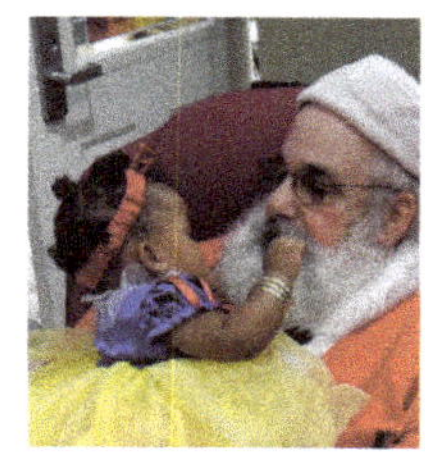

Michael J. Sanders
November 28, 1953–June 16, 2022

Mike was no storefront Santa with a fake beard and a pillow tucked under his jacket. Mike intentionally grew his beard all year long so it would be soft and snuggly for the little ones he held in his arms. The sack Santa Mike carried was very real too. This bundle of gifts he had flung on his back were given by God so that Mike could give back.

The first box was enormous and overflowed with Mike's *kindness, friendship* and *love.* Mike was bigger than life and he lovingly shared his heart.

A box marked *Servant* was laden with purpose. Mike served in the United Sates Air Force, where he willingly cared for our great nation.

Michael loved the Lord and served selflessly at Village View Community Church in Summerfield, Florida. There, he facilitated DivorceCare for over ten years providing support, encouragement, and healing for those who were lost and hurting.

His Santa ministry reached out to those in civic organizations and far into the community. Some of his elves came from Buffalo, NY to share the joy at Village View's yearly Fall Festivals. He ministered to and loved thousands.

In January 2022, Mike's spiritual commitment led him to become a church leader on the Elder Advisory Board.

The biggest gift in his pack was marked *"Giver of Care".*

Michael was a caregiver, not for a family member, he chose to be a caregiver for his 94-year-old neighbor. They bantered back and forth, but they loved each other, and Mike was heartbroken when she died.

Finally, it was *Jesus* that opened the last box in Santa's bag. There was an envelope in it, and a note that read *"Michael J. Sanders, an exceptional man and an exceptional child of God."*

Contents

Words of Introduction

A word of welcome

Let me be the first to welcome you to a safe place to share your feelings, stories, challenges and blessings, a place where relationships are made, growth is achieved, and God is present.

This *Journey Guide* can be used for groups or individual study.

A word of vision

Many caregiver groups are limited to member sharing and support.

I believe a better approach is the combination of learning opportunities, the assurance of God's love, and application of the *Moment-Method*, a way for caregivers and their loved ones to add meaning and joy on their difficult path.

A word for groups and individuals

Our lives are so often overwhelming, we all yearn for an ideal time when situations and relationships could be the way we imagine they should be. "When troubles of any kind come your way, consider it an opportunity for great joy" (James 1:2 NLT).

The text *Moments that Matter; a roadmap for caregivers and their loved ones with memory loss* and this *Journey Guide* will lead you to rich and life-changing opportunities.

A word for facilitators

You are the ones God has chosen to lead this support group. There is a GPS (GROUP Positioning System) in this journey guide for you. Contact me at www.moment-making.com to receive additional help, encouragement, and answers to any questions.

A word of inspiration

Caregivers, as you follow this roadmap you will begin to understand that caregiving is an act of worship—your spirit responding to God's spirit. The road is rough, you will face uncharted territories, detours and heartache, but know that you are giving God glory with every step you take.

A word of gratitude

Thank you to my husband, Donald, for his unending love, support and encouragement.

Praying that you and your loved one walk in the love of Jesus
as you bring a new focus to your journey.

Karen

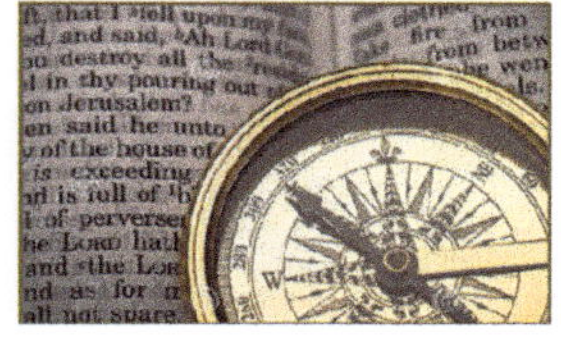

How to Navigate the Journey Guide

Turning to the Word of God
Follow the caregiver path with Scripture and God's love.

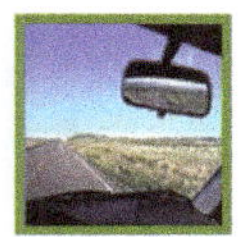

Expanding your horizons
Learning opportunities for caregivers and their loved ones

"Dears" Crossing: reflection and discussion

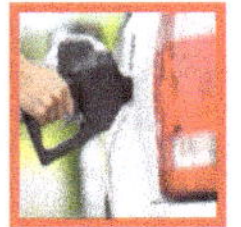

Care for the caregiver
Ways to keep your gas tank full

Journey Guide Answer Key
Appendix

At-Home Study

Prepare for future meetings. Read *MTM BOOK*. Apply journey concepts. Completing the At-Home Study will make the group sessions more productive.

Welcome to Your Caregiver Journey

Introductions… Guidelines… Benefits

A Bible-Based Presentation
Learning Opportunities… Encouragement… Enlightenment

BENEFITS OF THIS CAREGIVER SUPPORT GROUP:

- Receive needed support and scriptural encouragement.

- Learn applicable information, tools, and techniques.

- Learn why *Care for the caregiver* is so important.

- Together, caregivers grow stronger. When you share your caregiver journey and your personal input, you help yourself and others to grow.

- Gain knowledge about memory loss. Factually, in the future, you will have someone in your life that will benefit greatly from your education in this area.

- The main benefit of this caregiver support group is to learn how to make *moments* that will bring JOY to the journey of caregivers and their loved ones.

> We are the boat people, no two caregivers are alike and no two journeys are alike, yet, WE ARE ALL IN THE SAME BOAT!

We will all face an incredible challenge. Together, we will learn, support, encourage, and share our stories, successes, and challenges. We will pray for the group and for each person's individual journey.

In Appendix B, you will find a BOAT page that is to be copied and cut into three separate cards: spiritual bookmark, affirmation boat card, and caregiver scripture verse.

Spiritual Bookmark

Then he got into the boat and his disciples followed him. Without warning, a furious storm came up on the lake, so the waves went over the boat. But Jesus was sleeping. The disciples went and woke him saying, "Lord we are going to drown!" He replied, "You of little faith, why are you so afraid?" Then he got up and rebuked the wind and the waves, and it was completely calm. The men were amazed and asked, "What kind of man is this? Even the wind and waves obey him." (Matthew 8:23–27 NIV)

We learn in this passage that we, as caregivers, can have peace knowing that when "caregiver storms" arise with fury, anger, and frustrations, we can go to Jesus. Even the wind and the waves obey him, and he will calm our storms. He will save us from drowning. Jesus is in our boat.

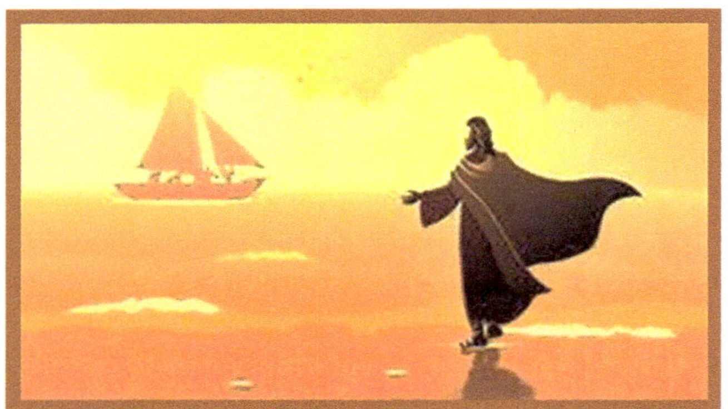

Affirmation Boat Card

Hang this affirmation card where you can see it often—on the mirror, dashboard, kitchen cabinet, etc. Each time you read it, you will be reminded that you are not alone. Seek God during hard times, and praise him on both good and bad days.

<h1 style="text-align:center">Caregiver Scripture Verse</h1>

A nightly reminder of God's promise:

"Come to me all you are weary and burdened, and I will give you rest."
(Matthew 11:28 NIV)

 **Turning to the Word of God**

Our caregiver scripture verse, Matthew 11:28, is a promise verse: When you come to him, he will give you rest. If you do your part, Jesus will do his.

Keep this verse by your bedside. Read and pray it each night, and it will comfort you. Allow Jesus to give you peace and rest after a long day and strength for a new day to come.

We are reassured and encouraged that caring for the sick glorifies God by reflecting our love for him. (Matthew 25:36–40 NIV).

Caregiving is an act of ___________________; your spirit responding to God's spirit, you will be ___________________ when you bring your best.

They are not giving you a hard time as much as they, themselves, are having a hard time.

> **At-Home Study**
>
> For future meeting, read *MTM BOOK*, pages 9–10. Begin using your three cards: affirmation boat card, scripture verse card, and bookmark.

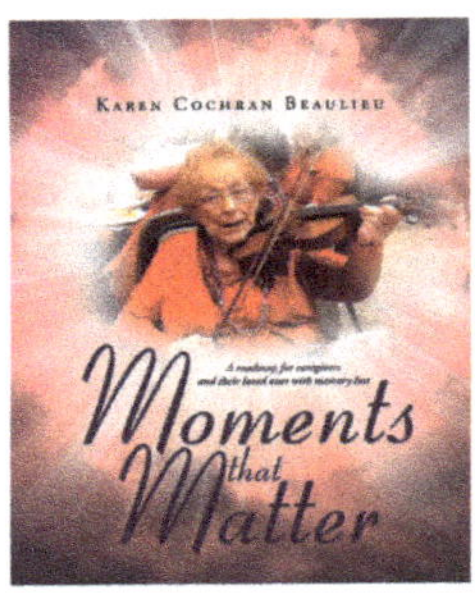

The texts: *Moments that Matter; a roadmap for caregivers and their loved ones with memory loss* (*MTM*) and *Moments that Matter: Journey Guide* (*JG*)
Website: www.moment-making.com
Other online searches: Cochran Beaulieu—Amazon, Google, and YouTube (video)

Read aloud *MTM BOOK*, pages 14–15

The Stages of Dementia Chart. Determine how it pertains to your loved one. If your loved has a non-dementia illness that is causing memory loss, such as Huntington's Disease, Parkinson's Disease, brain injury, or other disabilities, research the stages of that illness.

The term dementia presents symptoms of many illnesses—Alzheimer's, Parkinson's Disease, Huntington's Disease, stroke, hearing and vision problems, depression, cancer, kidney disease, hormone or thyroid disorders, infections, prescription and surgical drugs, alcoholism, liver disease, urinary tract infections (UTI), blood clots, AIDS, Tourette's syndrome, physical disabilities, amnesia, autism, and other traumatic life events, such as surgery, hospitalizations, and falls.

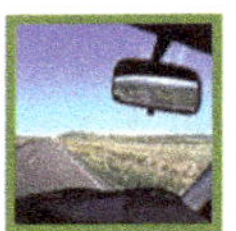 **Expanding your horizons**

Dementia is an umbrella term. What exactly is it? Read *MTM BOOK*, bottom of page 13.

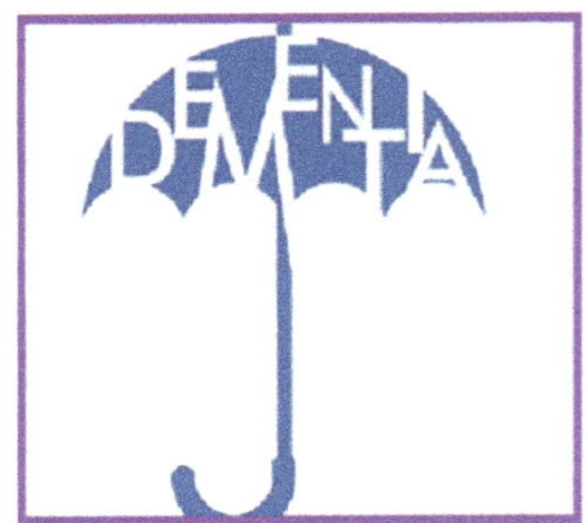

Alzheimer's disease is the largest and most common illness under the dementia umbrella, but there are many other illnesses that include memory loss, like those listed above. They present memory loss and dementia-like symptoms, some of which are irreversible and some are not.

Dementia begins _______________________, followed by a continual _______________________ that significantly impairs the ability to make decisions, perform personal care tasks, work, and successfully continue with social interactions and relationships.

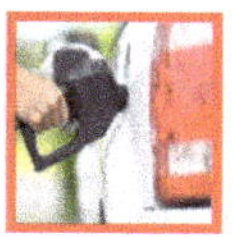

Care for the caregiver

Caregivers, have you ever, sometimes or quite often, especially on your most frustrating days, asked yourself the following questions?

- Why am I doing this?

- Does anyone appreciate what I'm doing?

- Why me?

If you answered *yes* to these questions, don't feel guilty. We as boat people have probably all felt this way at one time or another. You are not alone! If your answer was *no* or *sometimes*, that is perfectly fine too.

All three answers can be emotionally heartbreaking for the caregiver. **Read aloud** the heartfelt poem on *MTM BOOK*, page 11. It is a true reminder of why we do and what we do. *Share your feelings together about this poem.*

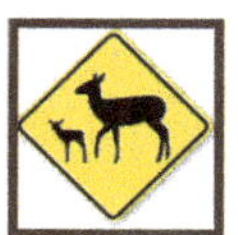

"Dears" Crossing: reflection and discussion

Read aloud "A Birthday Moment," *MTM BOOK*, pages 18–19.

What were some of the problems with Jonathan's big-impact-party approach and his understanding of his mother's illness?

Have you ever experienced this way of thinking in your situation? How?

It is the caregiver's job to _____________________ about their loved one's illness and to change their way of thinking, since the loved one has no control over their changes. Relationships will strengthen and cause less frustration and stress when you replace _____________________ with _____________________. This presents an extremely difficult challenge for the caregiver. Be gentle and patient with yourself during this process.

 **Turning to the Word of God**

"Have I not commanded you? Be strong and courageous. Do not be afraid: do not be discouraged: for the Lord your God will be with you wherever you go." (Joshua 1:9 NIV)

Share your thoughts about how this scripture can be an encouragement as caregivers make personal changes. When caregivers have a willingness to accept the illness and change _____________________, both they and their loved ones will become less frustrated and can move forward toward better lives.

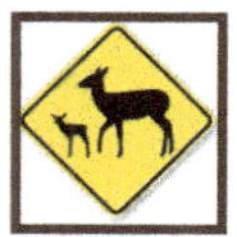

"Dears" Crossing: reflection and discussion

Consider ways you might change the way you think, the way you react, and the way you love. Brainstorm and record some possible next steps for caregivers, What might be your personal next step? If you commit to an action plan it will become a fruitful habit.

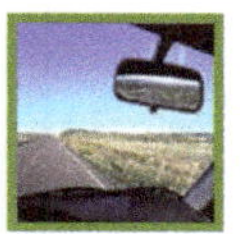

Expanding your horizons

Read aloud "Early Dementia Symptoms," *MTM BOOK*, bottom of pages 39–40, and the *10 Warning Signs of Alzheimer's.*

Ten warning signs of Alzheimer's (Alzheimer's Association):

1. Memory loss

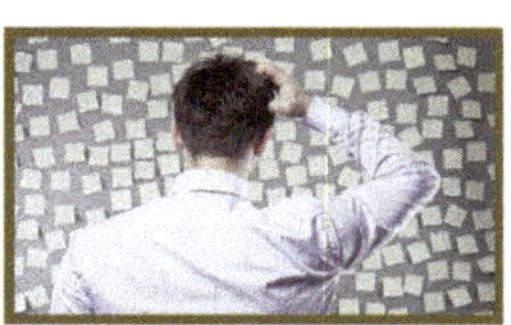

It's natural to occasionally forget an assignment, a deadline, or a person's name, but frequent forgetfulness or unexplainable confusion at home or in the workplace may signal something is wrong.

2. Difficulty performing familiar tasks

Busy people get distracted from time to time. For example, you might leave something on the stove for too long or not remember to serve part of a meal. People with Alzheimer's might prepare a meal and not only forget to serve it but also forget they made it.

3. Problems with language

Everyone has trouble finding the right word sometimes, but a person with Alzheimer's may forget simple words or substitute inappropriate words, making sentences difficult to understand.

4. Disorientation to time and place

It's normal to momentarily forget the day of the week or what you need from the store. People with Alzheimer's can become lost on their own streets, not knowing where they are, how they got there, or how to get back home.

5. Poor or decreased judgment

Choosing not to bring a sweater along on a chilly night is a common mistake. A person with Alzheimer's, however, may dress inappropriately in more noticeable ways, wearing a bathrobe to the store or several blouses on a hot day.

6. Problems with abstract thinking

Balancing a checkbook can be challenging for many people, but for someone with Alzheimer's, recognizing numbers or performing basic calculations may be impossible.

7. Misplacing things

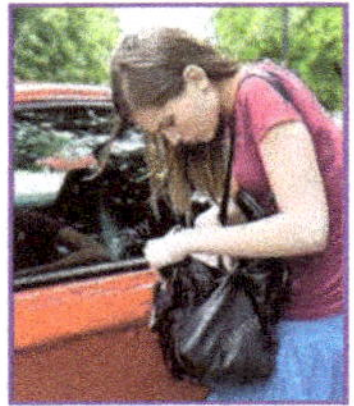

Everyone temporarily misplaces a wallet or keys from time to time. A person with Alzheimer's disease may put items in inappropriate places—such as an iron in the freezer or a wristwatch in a sugar bowl—and they have no recollection of how they got there.

8. Changes in mood or behavior

Everyone experiences a broad range of emotions—it's part of being human. People with Alzheimer's tend to exhibit more-rapid mood swings for no apparent reason.

9. Changes in personality

People's personalities may change somewhat as they age, but a person with Alzheimer's can change dramatically, either suddenly or over a period of time. Someone who is generally easygoing may become angry, suspicious, or fearful.

10. Loss of initiative

It's normal to tire of housework, business activities, or social obligations, but most people retain or eventually regain their interest. The person with Alzheimer's' disease may remain disinterested and uninvolved in many or all of their usual pursuits.

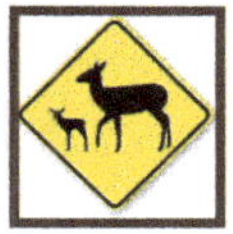 ## "Dears" Crossing: reflection and discussion

As you read about these beginning stages of memory loss, did you recognize any of these symptoms in your own behavior?

Did you ever go into a room and wonder why you were there? Have you ever not been able to think of a word in the middle of a conversation? Do you spend a lot of time looking for misplaced items? Do you ever have trouble doing something that is seemingly easy? Have you ever found that you put an unusual item in the refrigerator?

Mostly, as we age, these symptoms will show up occasionally. Usually, they just happen when we are tired, multitasking, stressed out, burnt out, super busy, or overwhelmed with the business of living life. Maintaining healthy lives include a balance of rest, exercise, diet, and brain activities.

A Roadmap for Healthy Minds

Route 1
Challenge Your Brain

- Pursue hobbies that challenge you.
- Learn something new.
- Repeat things you want to memorize.
- Organize lists into groups.
- Create mental images that will boost your memory.
- Use brain-training apps.
- Postpone your brain's aging with memory challenges.
- Use compensatory skills.

Route 2
Enjoy Yourself

- Hang out with friends.
- Allow yourself to laugh.
- Read! Read! Read!
- Stay positive.
- Create memories that matter.
- Inventory what you enjoy.
- Keep a diary of events in your life.
- Create a legacy for your family.

Route 4
Deal with Stress

- Address what triggers your stress.
- Meditate daily.
- See a mental health professional.
- Monitor your "self-talk."
- Focus on capabilities, not deficits.
- Look to others for support.
- Simplify your world.
- Finish well in life.

Route 3
Stay Healthy

- Promote good health.
- Get plenty of sleep.
- Eat brain-healthy foods.
- Drink brain-healthy beverages.
- Choose complex carbs.
- See your doctor regularly.
- Watch for medications that interact with each other.

Dr. Joanne Pitera Studer, Licensed Psychologist

If any of these signs did apply to you, what feelings and/or concerns might you have? What are some solutions that might make your life less busy and stressful?

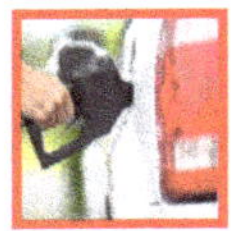 ## Care for the caregiver

Read and consider *Dr. Jo's Healthy Mind Chart, JG*, pages 10–11. Choose one or two items on the chart, and add them to your schedule.

Group member challenge. Become encouragement-accountability partners by periodically asking your fellow group members, "How are things going?" or "What would motivate you?" with their new health-plan choices. This is an excellent way to help each other to form new habits.

As these changes are achieved, continue to add other healthy choices to your lifestyle. Your challenging journey as a caregiver will be much easier when you are healthy.

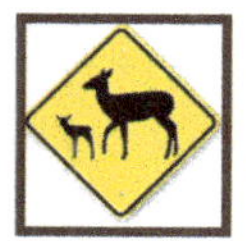

"Dears" Crossing: reflection and discussion

Read *The Stages of Dementia Chart, MTM BOOK,* pages 14–15. After you reviewed the dementia stages chart or researched your loved one's illness as part of your last At-Home Study, did the symptoms of their memory loss or other condition become clearer? How?

How did this increase your understanding of your role as a caregiver?

Regardless of specific illnesses, an _____________________ of each stage and symptom is an important tool in understanding the caregiver/loved one relationship.

Many people with dementia, depending on the stage of their illness, live their lives within specific time frames. They are able to enjoy activities, events, and gatherings but are not able to remember specifics either before or after the event.

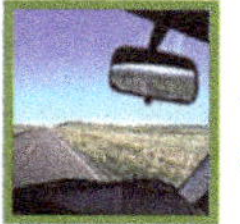

Expanding your horizons

Moments: *MTM BOOK,* pages 16–21.

What is a moment?

A _____________________ _____________________ between a caregiver and a loved one.

The creation of *Moments that Matter* for you and your loved one is the most important quality of life concept that a caregiver will ever need.

Moment Components

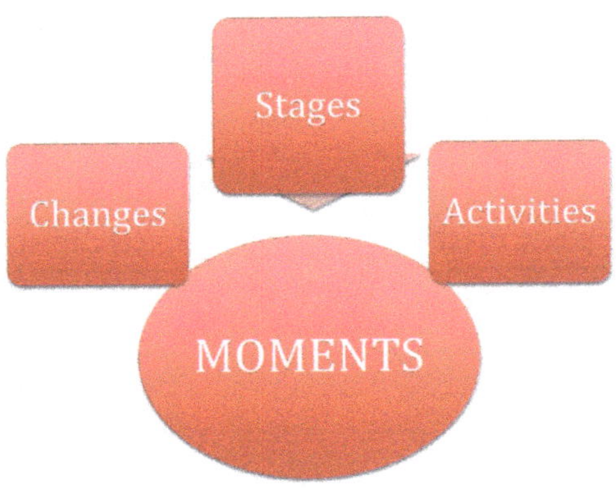

There are _____________________ components to moment-making. **Component 1** is changes and **Component 2** is stages.

Every journey and illness will present differently, so individual consideration and observation of your loved one's changes (component 1) and stages symptoms (component 2) are extremely important.

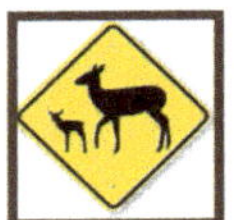 **"Dears" Crossing: reflection and discussion**

Consider the following changes and stages that are specific to your situation and your loved one's ability to perform the following tasks:

- Cognitive (changes in thinking or reasoning)

- Physical changes

- Behavioral changes

- Emotional changes

Which of these changes are hardest for you as a caregiver and why? Which of these changes do you believe are the hardest for your loved one?

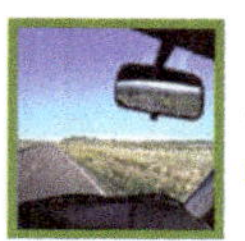

Moments: *MTM BOOK*, pages 16–21. **Component 3** is an enjoyed activity.

The most important goal of a moment will be if your loved one is _____________________ and doing something they enjoy.

Caregivers should always choose activities that are age and ability appropriate for their loved one's memory-loss stage. What brings them joy? When choosing activities, focus on their preferences, not busyness. If they did not enjoy puzzles before their illness symptoms occurred, they will not enjoy them now.

Many activity categories and examples are presented in detail in the *MTM BOOK*, pages 73–125. All journeys are unique, so careful review of these activities by the caregiver is key and will help with the creation of *everyday moments*. Encourage family, friends, and children to participle in moment-making as they can provide joy for everyone involved.

When does a moment really matter?

When all three of the following questions are answered:

What can they do?   *What do they need?*   *What do they like?*

Application of the *Moment-Method* is a simple way to create quality time with your loved one. Many of these *everyday moments* will become favorites and can be used again and again. An example would be looking at the same photo albums together more than once.

Meaningful connections will improve quality of life for you and your loved one when all _____________________ components are used.

Read aloud *MTM BOOK*, pages 16–17.

What isn't a moment?

When an attempted connection is not made. This happens when one or more moment _____________________ are missing.

Can a moment be saved?

Yes, try the activity again and use all three components correctly.

> "Quality time together…trumps time together"
>
> (Alzheimer's Association).

At-Home Study

Using the "Moment Components" in *MTM BOOK*, page 19, try creating an *everyday moment that matters*, once a week, until your group meets again. Consider activity ideas, *MTM BOOK*, pages 75–125.

Note: Focus on things that your loved one enjoys and remembers and not *what you think should* be enjoyed and remembered, *MTM BOOK*, page 17.

 **Turning to the Word of God**

"The Lord will guide you always, he will satisfy your needs in a sun-scorched land and will strengthen your frame." (Isaiah 58:11 NIV)

Pray that God will guide your time spent together and that it brings happiness to both you and your loved one.

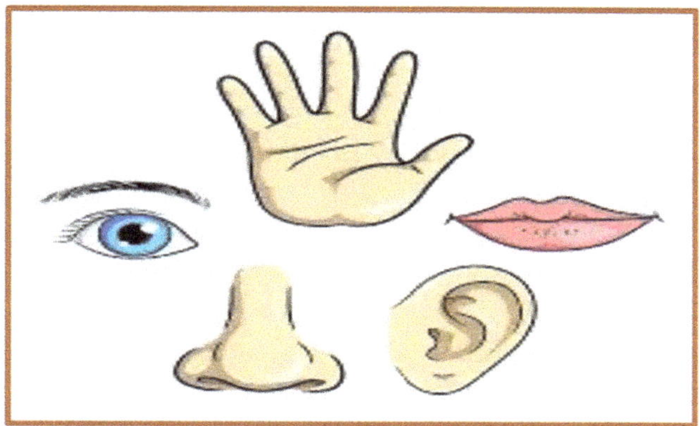

Read aloud *MTM BOOK*, page 24, "A Family Christmas" and the following paragraph, and *MTM BOOK*, page 20, "Tutu and Tails" and the following paragraph.

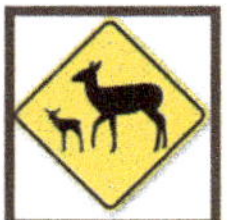 **"Dears" Crossing: reflection and discussion**

How do the senses mentioned in these stories satisfy the three components of the *Moment-Method?*

Brainstorm ways that sensory components can be added to bring success to your moment making.

Sensory components don't require any ___________________ abilities on the part of the loved one. These are particularly recommended as successful activities for those in the declining stages of dementia. Share the successes and challenges you have experienced making *everyday moments*.

Sensory moments are a great opportunity for intergenerational gatherings with younger family members.

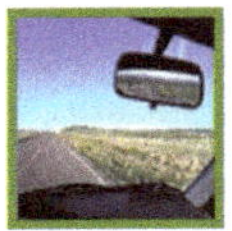 ## Expanding your horizons

Grand moments: *MTM BOOK*, page 23. We are now familiar with the three components of the *Moment-Method* illustrated in the *MTM BOOK*, page 19, that are needed to make *everyday moments*.

This method is also used to create *grand moments*, ones that make a strong impression because of their greatness, dignity, and/or splendor. They require ___________________ ___________________ on the part of the caregiver, so getting assistance from family and friends is suggested.

Read aloud the following two examples of *grand moments*. Ever wonder about the woman on the front cover of the *Moments that Matter* book? Allow me to introduce my mother, Betty. Her story, "The Face in the Photograph," *MTM BOOK*, page 26, is an example of her *grand moment*.

This is a true moment, one that gave great joy to me, as her daughter and caregiver, and was especially meaningful to her. It was a moment that truly mattered.

The second *grand moment* story is "Empty Vines," *MTM BOOK*, page 25. This is also a true story, and it brought great joy to him and his family.

Reliving these grand moments with your loved one using photo memories presents a bonus activity for reminiscing and conversation. It becomes a useful technique for

______________________ ______________________.

In the reality of your loved one with memory loss, seeing photographs will present each time as a new experience and thus can be an enjoyable moment over and over again.

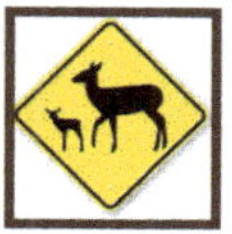 ## "Dears" Crossing: reflection and discussion

We have learned what moments are and what they are not. We have learned how to save a failing moment. We have learned an effective method to create *everyday* and *grand moments*. We have learned that creating intentional and successful moments brings joy to loved ones, caregivers, family, and friends.

Making *moments* is the crux of a positive approach to caregiving. Review the *grand moment* ideas on *MTM BOOK*, pages 24–25. Holiday Tips are in Appendix C.

Which of these examples might be used in the future with you and your loved one?

When these moment-making skills and techniques are applied to your caregiver journey, your job will become easier, and you will see improvement in the quality of life of your loved one.

 ## Turning to the Word of God

"Now that you know these things you will be blessed if you do them."
(John 13:17 NIV)

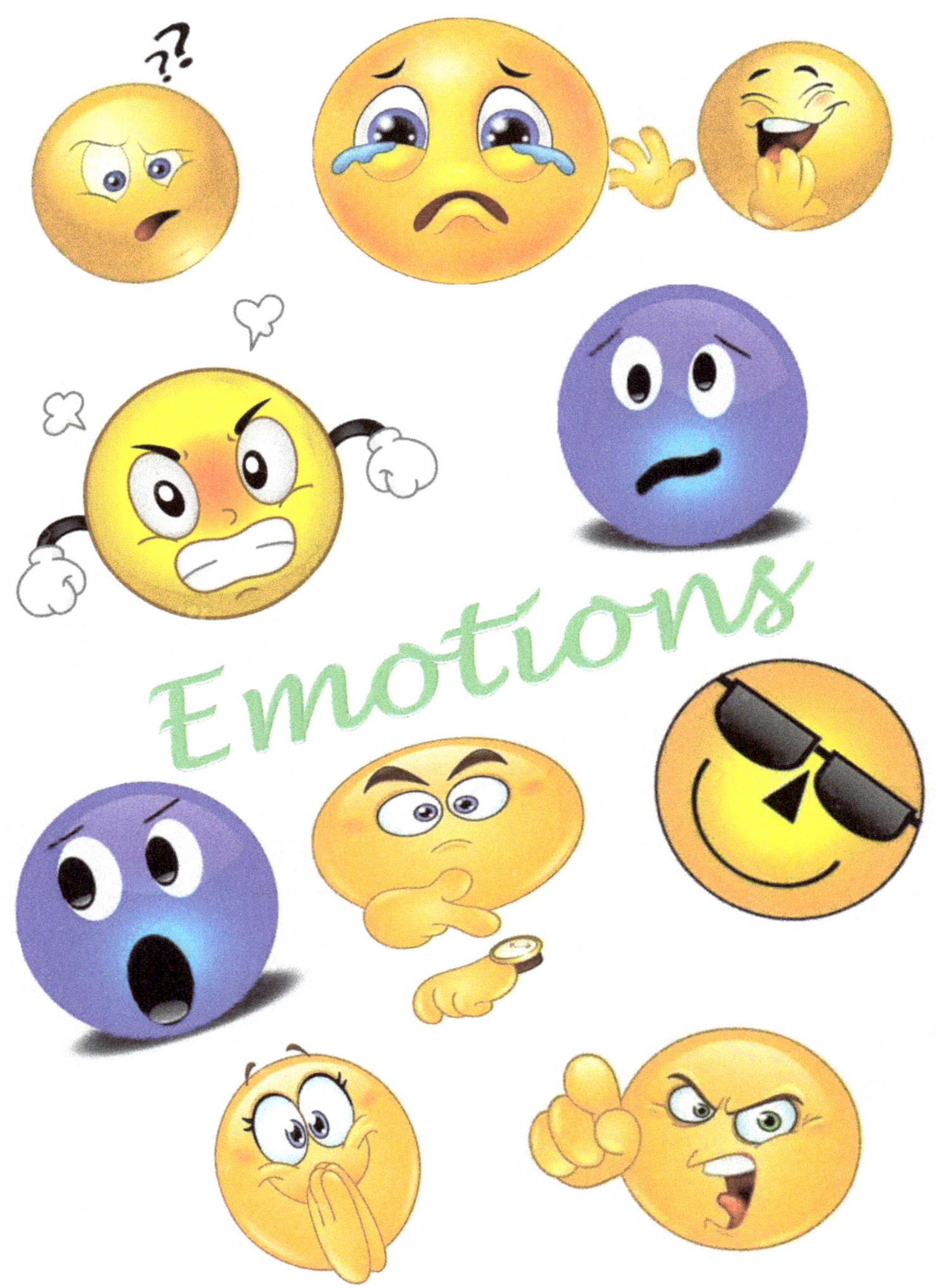
Emotions

Caregiver Emotions: What's Rocking Our Boat?

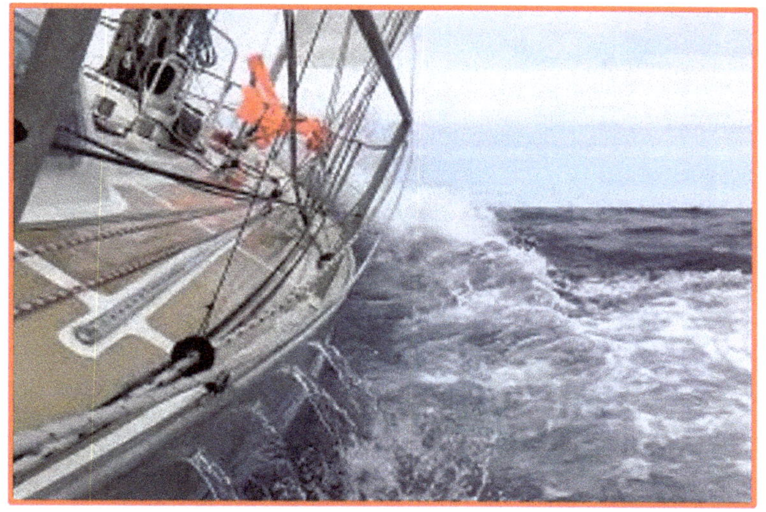

Group members: Individually pick the two emotions that best represent your life as a caregiver, and share together why you chose them.

Emotions affect the journey of both the caregiver and their loved ones. What does the rhythm of your life look like?

It is normal and expected that many challenging emotions and heartaches will arise on the caregiver journey. It can be sometimes like a seesaw, a hamster's wheel, or a Whack-A-Mole game. The good news is that our great God is the one with the hammer!

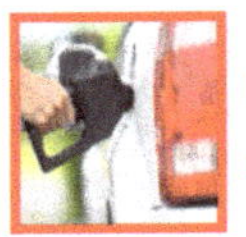

Care for the caregiver

Unfortunately, negative emotions left ___________________ can sometimes grow into heightened negative emotions.

- "This is too hard" can change to hopelessness and feeling trapped.

- "I can't do this" can change to extreme frustration.

- "Why is this happening to me?" can change to helplessness and feelings of being totally overwhelmed.

- "I hate my life, and I am a horrible caregiver" can change to depression.

If you feel that any of these heightened emotions pertain to you, consider consulting pastoral care, counseling, senior services, in-home assistance, and/or hospice care.

Turning to the Word of God

Jesus can calm the wind and the waves! He is in our caregiver boat! Reminder: read your scripture bookmark every day. (Matthew 8:23–27 NIV). We are stronger when we support each other and rely on God's power and love.

Emotions Drama

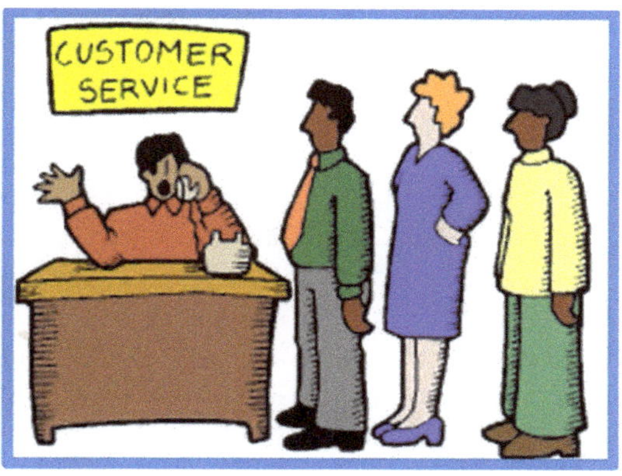

Choose two group members to participate, one to play the role of the sales associate and the other to play the role of the caregiver customer.

The Customer Service Counter

Sales Associate: "Hello, my name is Jesus. How can I help you today?"

Caregiver: "Hi, I have two things I would like to return for an even exchange."

Sales Associate: "What is the reason for these exchanges?"

Caregiver: "They just didn't fit me right. They were *way too* BIG for me! So I am returning ANGER. Please exchange it for JOY, and I am returning FRUSTRATION. Please exchange it for PEACE! Oh, and I would like both PEACE and JOY in a size five times or bigger!"

Sales Associate: "Certainly, you came to the right place; it is always our SOUL GOAL to make our customers joyful. We are happy to exchange Satan's emotional bees for God's Words of honey and healing."

Sales Associate: "Here's your receipt, and here is a free coupon for guidance, wisdom, and love with no expiration date! Also, please take a moment to go to our website, **way. truth.life.com**, and fill out the Customer Service Experience Survey. The BOSS likes to know how his sales associates are performing! Again, my name is Jesus. Thank you, and have a blessed day!"

Jesus offers an exchange system. Go from stressed to blessed!

At-Home Study

Using the *Moment Components*, *MTM BOOK*, page 19, try creating an *Everyday Moment that Matters*, once a week, until your group meets again. Consider activity ideas, *MTM BOOK*, pages 75–125.

Note: focus on things that your loved one enjoys and remembers and not <u>what you think should</u> be enjoyed and remembered, **MTM BOOK, page 17**.

Our Loved One's Emotions: What's Rocking Their Boat?

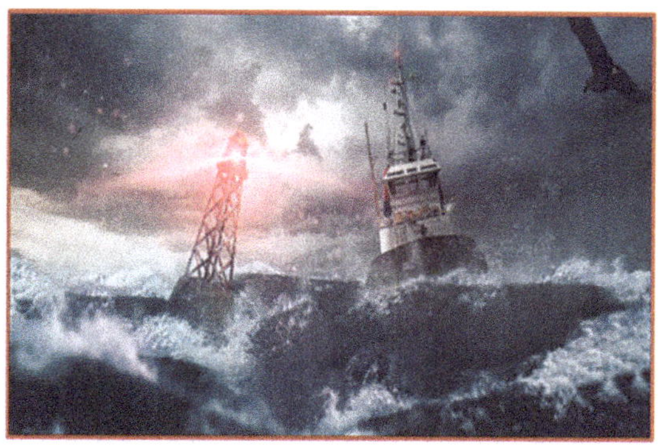

Read aloud "Seize the Day," *MTM BOOK*, page 36.

Sharon is seventy-two years old and has early dementia. Her husband passed away five years ago, and she lives alone.

What struggles did Sharon experience with her neighbor and friend?

Allow yourself to jump into Sharon's reality and experience the truths of cognitive impairment. Then consider these questions:

- Why did her emotions change?

- What new emotions did these become?

- How did her feelings change when the solicitor called?

Her cognitive frustrations were removed!

Did you, as Sharon, use reasoning skills to answer these questions?

We take thinking for granted!

You can't reason with someone who can't reason. Caregivers must learn to remove cognitive frustration for their loved ones.

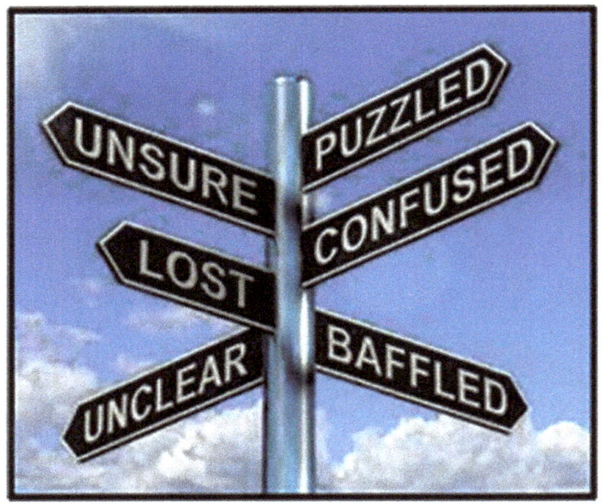

At-Home Study

Caregiver challenge: Catch yourself asking questions or making statements that require your loved one to reason.

Review Philippians 4:8. Write it down. Read it often. Intentionally focus on these positive words.

For future meeting, read *MTM BOOK*, pages 34–35, "The Big Jump."

"Dears" Crossing: reflection and discussion

What are some specific situations when you have asked your loved one to reason, without considering that this mental task was a difficult or an impossible thing for them to do? When recalling these situations, what emotions or behaviors did they exhibit?

Caregivers are the ones that must continually change their approach because those with dementia _____________________ control their changes.

Turning to the Word of God

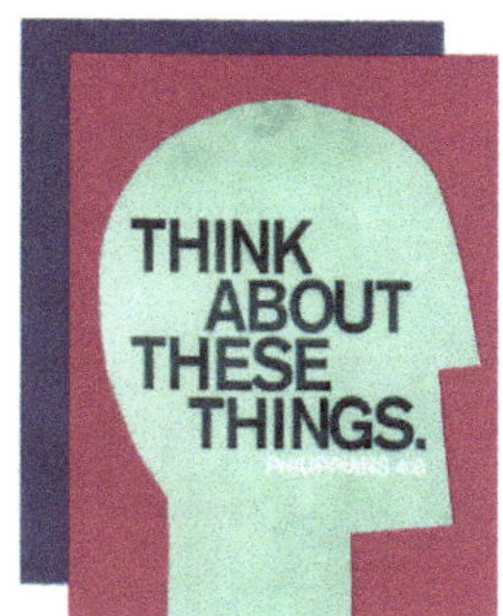

"Finally brothers and sisters, whatever is *true*, whatever is *noble* whatever is *pure*, whatever is *lovely*, whatever *is admirable*—if anything is *excellent* or *praiseworthy*—think about such things." (Philippians 4:8 NIV)

What we think about is what we become. As we intentionally add positive thought patterns to our life, we will begin to see changes and can expect:

- To worry and to have less stress

- To have an improved prayer life

- To see God's glory

- To have a renewed heart for the beauty of our loved one

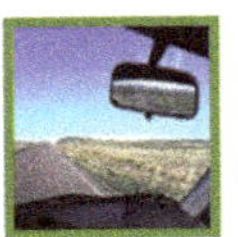

Expanding your horizons

The caregiver and their person are not living in the same reality.

Read Aloud "A Big Jump," *MTM BOOK*, page 34. This is a simple example of what I refer to as *reality jumping*. This is a way for caregivers to choose decisions based on things that might trigger their loved one's balance.

Situations that hurt and irritate them can be avoided when caregivers change their mindset. Allow them to make choices whenever possible and honor those choices. This will provide ____________________ - ____________________ in their world of lost dignity.

When a caregiver practices reality jumping, it allows their loved one's inner balance to be maintained and further ____________________ can be avoided.

As cognitive decline progresses, we must learn to adapt and accept symptoms and ability changes. Quality of life for everyone is always the goal, but along the way, caregivers will sometimes have to make decisions based on the fact that they know their choice is the only correct one.

Another antidote for reversing bad emotional behavior is laughter. Sometimes, spoken words, funny reactions, or behaviors will just give cause to burst out laughing. Saying to your person in a positive way, "Oh you are so funny," will allow you to laugh with them and not at them.

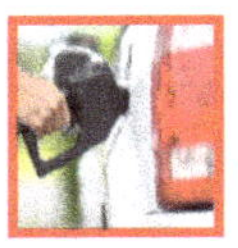

Care for the caregiver

Always strive to make ____________________ and joy be part of your caregiver journey. Laughter is a super stress reliever! Why and how should laughter be integrated into your journey?

- Laughter improves the overall quality of life, enhances learning abilities, and provides a wellness plan for your mind, body, and spirit. Consider these activities.

- Make a list of things that make you laugh, and put it in your daily routine.

- Put old and new comedy movies on your calendar. Invite friends and family to join you for a fun event. Don't forget the popcorn.

- Buy an ability- and age-appropriate joke or riddle book—share the ones you like or just "crack yourself up."

- A smile is contagious. Be a carrier by intentionally smiling at someone five times each day.

- Ask your family and friends to share funny stories or jokes with you and your loved one by phone, text, or during visits.

- Look for humor in serious situations. Get a clown nose. It will bring a smile every time.

- When your loved one needs a lift, put the big red nose on and casually walk into the room.

- When you need a lift, put it on, and go look in the mirror!

> **Humor and laughter can be integrated into a whole persons' wellness plan that can translate into improvements in your life: mind, body and spirit. (Bains)**

The Legacy of Deborah Wells

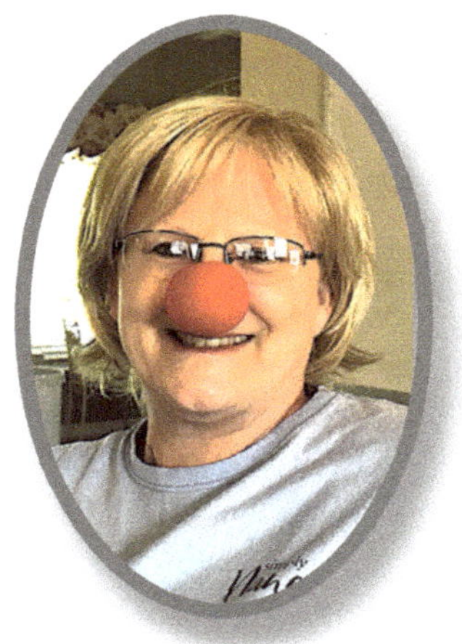

In Loving Memory
January 8, 1959–September 4, 2020

 During our caregiver support group in 2019, we all wore clown noses. Deborah learned to wear hers and use it as a therapeutic way to embrace laughter. She cheered the sad and even encouraged herself while facing the very demanding job of caregiving.

Deborah took a dozen of these clown noses and shared them with her fellow cancer patients and the nurses during their cancer chemo sessions.

During her illness, she posted a large copy of this picture on her refrigerator as a reminder to always find something to smile about while battling this painful disease. These smiling moments were created by her faithful relationship with Jesus and the great love she had for her family.

Unable to see her mother for months, Deborah sent her large "clown nose" photograph to her memory-care facility. It was lovingly placed so that her mom could see her daughter's smiling face every day.

 One of Deborah's last wishes was to share this picture at her Celebration of Life service. This is how she wanted to be remembered. She lived this legacy from deep within her heart and soul by spreading hope, love, and joy with her smiling face.

"Laughter is an instant vacation." (Milton Berle) 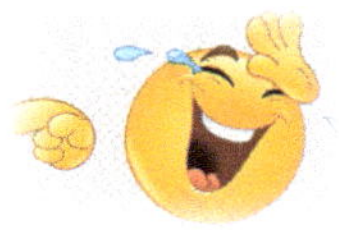

Did you know that you can't be _____________________ when you are laughing?

Our relationship with Jesus will always give us a reason to smile. Trust in him.

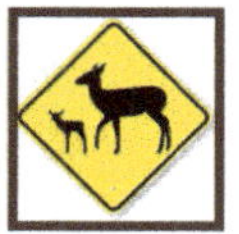 **"Dears" Crossing: reflection and discussion**

Consider and discuss the benefits of laughter in your life. What fun activities can be added to your caregiver situation?

Clearly, we can't face every situation with laughter. However, when we are discouraged and frustrated, we can reflect on how Jesus can calm the wind and the waves and that he is the center of our caregiver boat.

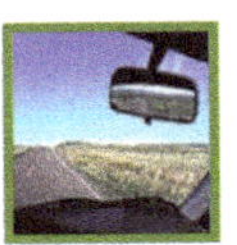

Expanding your horizons

Environment 1

A thorough consideration of your person's environment will provide safety, stimulation, and visual activity.

As we review *MTM BOOK*, pages 49–52, we learn that _________________ is the most important of the senses because most of the information we receive is acquired by sight stimulation.

When vision problems and dementia join forces, much greater difficulties are created. The most common are blurred vision, loss of peripheral vision, and altered color perception.

Visual appreciation is acquired by bursts of color seen in sparkling decorations, brilliant colors in nature, and bright interiors in the environment. Colors have the ability to calm, stimulate, and make rooms appear larger and smaller.

> **At-Home Study**
>
> **For future meeting**, read *MTM BOOK*, pages 55–58, "Memory Techniques."

Turning to the Word of God

The Bible tells us in Genesis that God created the heavens and the earth and his spirit hovered over it all and made everything good. He then created light, oceans, and sunshine. He created all the different trees, flowers, and all of nature. He made everything beautiful to give pleasure to his children.

It is not at all surprising to me that God provided a way for those with aged eyes and cognitively diminished minds to maintain the ability to appreciate his beautiful creations.

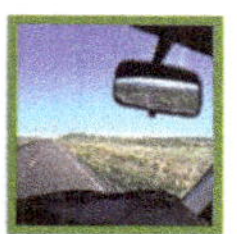

Expanding your horizons

Environment 2

Below are excerpts taken from "Environmental Changes," *MTM BOOK*, pages 52–54. They show examples of environmental safety, color and perception.

- Colors awaken emotional responses, increase or decrease visibility, and can make environments bright and beautiful.

- Bold contrast patterns on floors and carpeting can cause ____________________ and confusion. Black entry rugs and those with checkered patterns can be perceived as ____________________.

- Floors that lead into each other should be the ____________________ color. A tan bedroom rug leading into a tan-tiled bathroom floor would be a good choice.

- Avoid falls by using nonskid rugs, removing ill-placed electric cords, and fixing any uneven walkways.

- Aging eyes do not perceive subtle changes in carpets, steps, floors, and walls. This makes the world of memory loss more confusing and difficult.

"Dears" Crossing: reflection and discussion

Environment

Close your eyes, and mentally explore your loved one's living spaces.

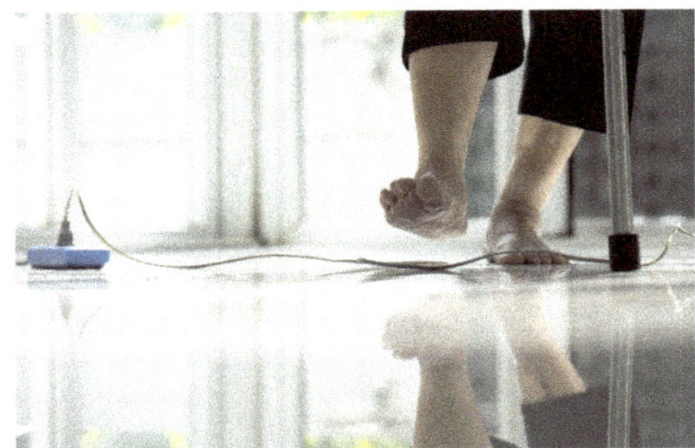

- Are there things that might present a safety issue?

- Are there colors that might improve stimulation and/or decrease emotional upset?

- Would high-contrast colors make your person's daily living easier?

- Are there interior pathways or carpets that need to be reconsidered?

Discuss any problem areas in your loved one's environment, and together, suggest ways to improve environmental spaces.

Make changes during the early stages of memory loss so ______________________ will be easier and confusion will be limited.

"Dears" Crossing: reflection and discussion

Memory Retention Techniques

Lifestyle changes that include memory techniques and enhancers are incredibly valuable in the task of retaining memories and information and prolonging _______________ ________________.

Review and share the following techniques and any other ways you know that will help retain memories, *MTM BOOK*, pages 55–58+.

Memory retention techniques:

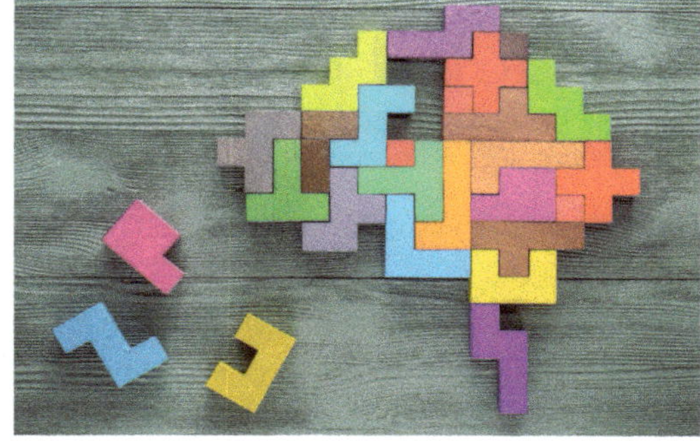

- The notebook

- Clocks and radios

- Games/puzzles

- Reminiscing

- Photo albums

- Reminder labels

- Whiteboards

- Phones

Search *Alzheimer's and dementia products* online for other suggestions.

Expanding your horizons

Communication 1

Communication is the key to success in the workplace, churches, relationships, and families. We have all experienced the overwhelming struggle of attaining and maintaining good communication.

According to Anne Converse Willkomm, there are five basic types of communication:

- Verbal: This includes speaking with others, how we string words together, the complexity of those words, and tone of voice. These conversations can be face-to-face or on any other communication devices.

- Nonverbal: These present as sharing ideas of feelings through facial expressions, posture, eye contact, hand movements, and touch.

- Written: These are communicated by email, mail, memo, note, or report.

- Listening: We cannot effectively communicate without listening. We must consider engagement and negotiation as part of each conversation.

- Visual communication: This includes receiving messages from photographs, television, Internet, Facebook, videos, books, etc.

The symptoms of cognitive decline add extremely difficult ______________________ for caregivers and their loved ones.

Confusion and agitation often result when memory impairment, loss of judgment, the ability to ___________________, and poor language skills exist.

Thus, it becomes harder for the caregiver to be patient, and this often results in ___________________ and poor self-esteem for the loved one. There are more sensitive ways to increase success in most communication situations.

Communication role-play challenge:

- You are deciding what to prepare for dinner. What would you say if you want your loved one to be included in choosing an entrée? (Limit choices to two.)

- You are ordering a meal at a restaurant. How would you help your person order from a menu? (Suggest two entrees you know they like.)

- You are having a conversation about something in the care receiver's past. (Using the key phrases "show me" and "tell me" can be used so that your loved one can successfully communicate without having to answer specific questions.)

- If your loved one's ability no longer allows them to mentally retrieve answers to short-term memory questions. (Communication with your loved one will be more successful if you ask "yes" or "no" questions?)

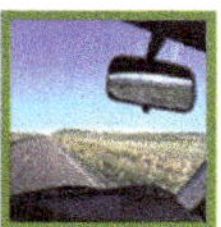 ## Expanding your horizons

Visiting stages and visiting words

Read aloud *MTM BOOK*, pages 42–44, and consider the stages and words for successful visiting.

Stages:

- Anticipation

- A complimentary greeting

- A planned activity

- An affectionate goodbye

These words should be used when visiting. Using affirmations is an especially good way for caregivers, family, and friends to communicate. In review, laughter has the power to build self-esteem for those with dementia. Try to keep your conversations light and upbeat when beginning or ending times together.

Sharing these communication skills in _________________ with expected visitors can make occasions and family gatherings more special.

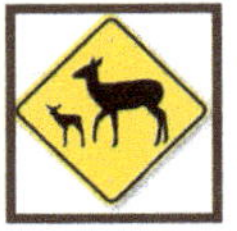 **"Dears" Crossing: reflection and discussion**

Read aloud the story "Hello Dolly," *MTM BOOK*, page 46.

How did Dolly try to cover her forgetfulness?

What similar ways have you noticed your person trying to hide their confusion?

How do these and other methods of communicating help to maintain dignity for those with dementia?

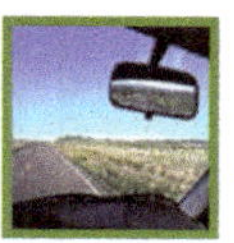

Expanding your horizons

Communication 2

According to Central Florida's Alzheimer's Family Organization, the following things are particularly difficult for those with cognitive impairment:

- Finding the right words

- Forgetting simple words

- Choosing the right words

- Being able to put a name to things and objects

- Verbal expression of wants and needs

- Problems with speaking, reading, and writing

- Ordering from a menu

- Money handling

- Checkout lines

- Places that are busy, loud, and colorful

> Ways to boost understanding:
>
> - Be as clear and specific as possible.
>
> - Use short sentences.
>
> - Give instructions one at a time.
>
> - Speak slowly.
>
> - Wait for nonverbal responses.
> (Spencer Scott)

As certain brain connections diminish, successful word processing often stops after the third word is heard. Your saying, "It's time for lunch" may cause frustration. Those with cognitive impairment may only hear the words "It's time for" and are confused about what you are saying. They usually will respond by saying, "What?" This response allows them to appear as if they have not heard the words rather than appear to be confused by the words. Using the three words "time for lunch" can be better understood. When speaking in sentences, it is better to pause after the third word, wait for the brain to process, and then speak three more words.

Turning to the Word of God

The Bible teaches us to use positive action words: *encourage, reassure, praise, complement, engage, include, share, love, listen, validate,* and *pray.*

Of course, we all will fail and revert to speaking _______________ words sometimes. A wise psalmist gives a prayer to use when our patience draws thin:

"Set a guard over my mouth, Lord, keep watch at the door of my lips."
(Psalm 141:3 NIV)

Although this task will always be a difficult work in progress for all of us, try taking a deep breath and repeating this Psalm before situations become heated.

"Dears" Crossing: reflection and discussion

Communication 3

What communication skills have been the most frustrating for you?

How can avoiding the use of pronouns in a conversation benefit a person's understanding?

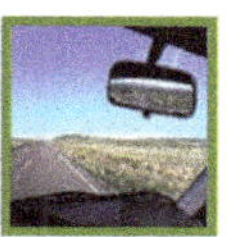

Expanding your horizons

Validation 1

What does validation mean?

- To confirm

- To verify

- To authenticate

- To support

- To endorse

Validation can be verbal or nonverbal. Validation requires an awareness of feelings followed by encouragement and understanding. Intentional focus on our loved one's feelings, frustrations, and discouragements is important for relational growth.

What is validation therapy? Validation therapy offers a holistic approach that empathizes with elderly patients and those with dementia by communication and connection. It was developed in the 1960s and 1970s by Naomi Feil. We still have a lot to learn from the human brain. Her validation method provides insight into the behaviors and thoughts of those who suffer from Alzheimer's disease and other types of dementia.

Trying to make an effort to communicate with those who have dementia, even though they may be disoriented and suffer from hallucinations, offers a practical way to help reduce their stress, enhance their dignity, and increase their happiness.

 ## Turning to the Word of God

Validation Skills

> "Be completely humble and gentle; be patient bearing with one another
> in love." (Ephesians 4:2 NIV)

Offering to _____________________ with your person is especially comforting and calming during these upsets.

> "Is anyone among you in trouble? Let them pray." (James 5:13 NIV)

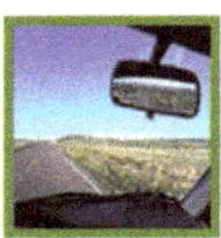 ## Expanding your horizons

Validation 2

Focus on listening and observing: if your person is upset, talking, or crying, nodding your head and holding their hand will validate them. (*Would you like to pray about it?*)

Focus on restating what the person is saying: if they are upset and complaining, use statements such as "You're thinking this is unfair and would like someone to listen to your viewpoint." (*Would you like to pray about it?*)

Focus on causes of behaviors including past and present: restate their past, and connect it to the present. "I remember this happened to you before, and it makes sense that it would upset you now." (*Would you like to pray about it?*)

This technique helps to restore confidence and dignity and helps us to gain some empathy for our loved one. It requires us to take time to ____________________ to them so that they can make us aware of where they are and what time frame they are referring to.

(Selsavage)
Added prayer suggestions (Cochran Beaulieu)

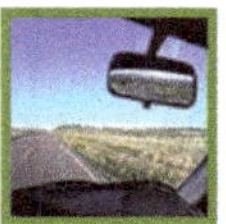 ## Expanding your horizons

Invalidation

What does invalidation mean?

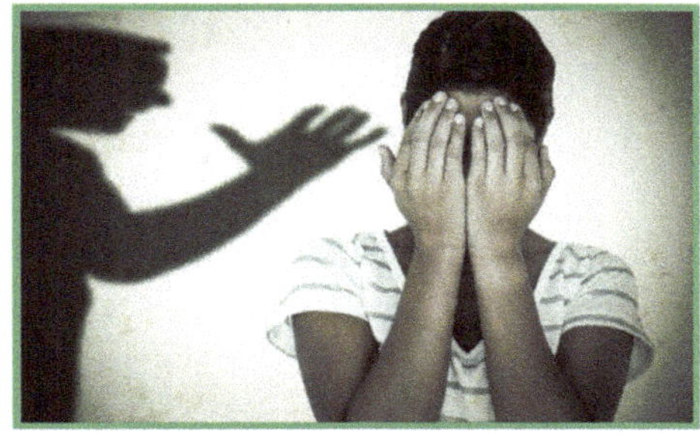

- To negate

- To dismiss behavior

What does invalidation do?

- Weakens

- Nullifies

- Cancels

- Ejects

Invalidation response examples

Reject self-description: Your loved one shares an experience that you know is not a true story.

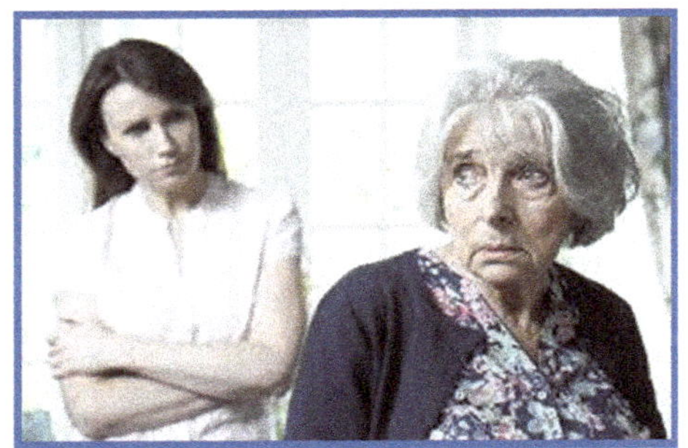

Caregiver response: "That didn't happen. You don't know what you are talking about."

Reject response to events as incorrect or ineffective: Your loved one says, "I'm such a burden to you."

Caregiver response: "Oh, Mom, it's stupid to feel that way."

Dismiss or disregard: Your loved one says, "I really miss my cat."

Caregiver response: "He was really old and lived a long time."

Directly criticize or punish: Your loved one spills her drink and makes a big mess.

Caregiver response: *Said with annoyance,* "Why can't you be more careful? I don't have time to clean that up!"

Reject and link responses to socially unacceptable characteristics: Your loved one bumps into a chair and begins to cry.

Caregiver response: "Oh for Pete's sake, you're alright. It's nothing to cry about.

How does invalidation affect us? It creates confusion, so we learn not to trust ourselves, and it tends to make us rely on others for the correct response.

It makes us ignore or repress our ______________________ and makes us extremely emotional. It causes us to view our failures, successes, and goals unrealistically.

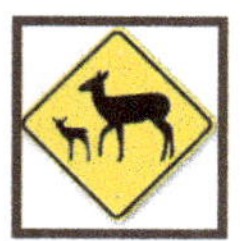 ## "Dears" Crossing: reflection and discussion

How do you feel when someone validates you?

Share some examples.

Has being invalidated ever changed the way you felt about yourself? How?

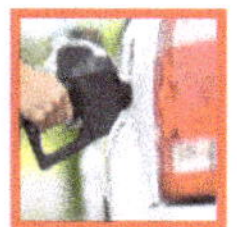 ## Care for the caregiver

Your weariness can be physical and/or emotional. Your burdens will be heavy. It is important to have a good ___________________ ___________________ in place to deal with feelings of hurt, guilt, frustration, and anger.

Remember to read our caregiver scripture verse, *JG*, page 3.

> "Come to me all you who are weary and burdened and I will give you rest." (Matthew 11:28 NIV)

Caregiving is an act of ___________________, your spirit responding to God's spirit. You will be blessed when you bring your best. Caregivers need to have people that support and validate them.

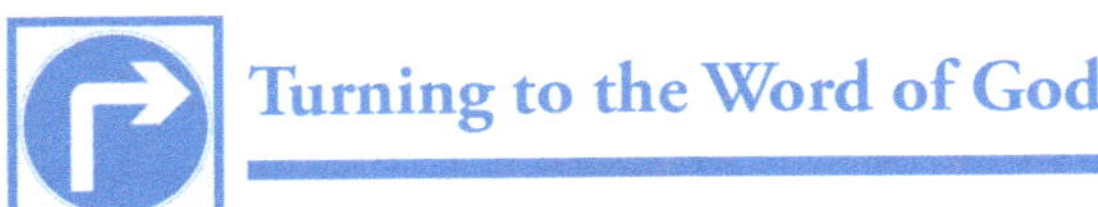

Turning to the Word of God

Honor means to regard with high respect, great esteem, and appreciation. Validation is the practice of honoring someone. The biblical emphasis on honoring others has everything to do with honoring God.

> "Love each other with genuine affection, and take delight in honoring each other." (Romans 12:10 NLT)

God will honor your efforts and multiply your blessings.

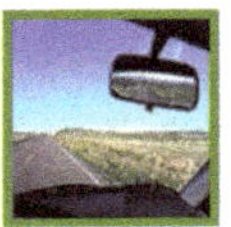

Expanding your horizons

Validation and Redirection

Redirection is the act of changing the course of conversation. This will immediately create a new thought pattern for the person with memory loss. It can be used successfully in many situations, and it is a must-needed tool for caregivers.

Much of our daily upset and annoyance will diminish by creating new conversations about a family member, an upcoming event, or even the weather whenever an upset occurs. How to use validation and redirection? **Read aloud** the following two examples.

Example 1: Although eighty years old, a woman with dementia may think that she is a teenager. An upset for her might occur when she desperately insists on going to her childhood home. She has become frantic with worry because her parents do not know her whereabouts.

Suggested response: To validate her upset, you might nod and say, "Oh, my dear, I understand how you might feel that your parents will be very concerned if you are late. I will go right now and see about calling them. I know they will be relieved to know you are safe.

Offer a quick prayer, and then ask her to sit down and relax. Smile and say, "I will be back to check on you in a few minutes."

When you return, use the redirection technique: "You look so pretty today. Let's go have a cup of tea together."

Example 2: Your uncle is looking for his wife and is becoming upset that he can't find her. He doesn't remember that she passed away years ago.

Suggested response: Don't try to correct him and tell him that his wife has passed away. This will certainly increase his upset. You can reply with a redirection statement, "I love Aunt Mary. Tell me about her." Allowing him to talk about his wife should lessen his fear and nervousness. By giving him the opportunity to reminisce, you have redirected his focus to another place.

"By using the words "tell me" or "show" me, you are acknowledging that they are not right or wrong. We must listen and observe what does and doesn't work with our loved one. Let them be the teacher. Allow them to educate us, and as long as we listen, we can learn from them. A person living with memory loss wants to feel normal and wants to fit in. They do not want to be corrected or to be made to look stupid or out of place. _______________________ can be used successfully for many situations. It is especially helpful in the afternoon when confusion may be an issue for your loved one." (Selsavage)

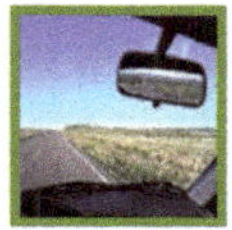

Expanding your horizons

Invalidation behaviors: "Why did they do that?"

As illness progresses, caregivers will see unusual behaviors. These are exhibited by changes in our loved one's personality and can be uncharacteristic and inappropriate.

These behaviors and words are a plea for help, understanding, and love.

Date yourself for a moment, and recall when VCR tapes were rented at video stores. The movie renter was always requested to BE KIND…REWIND.

Each behavior your person presents is their way of communicating what they want, what they need, or how they feel. It is up to the caregiver to investigate, find the _________________________________, and respond accordingly.

Ask the Holy Spirit to help and guide you as you realize these triggers. Think of your loved one's current life as a movie when a strange behavior occurs.

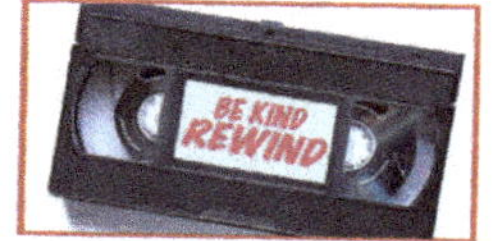

BE KIND…REWIND.

Roll back the tape until you discover what triggered the behavior. Most behaviors fall into one of these three modes:

- ___________________________

- ___________________________

- ___________________________

Fright mode: This behavior mode is often exhibited when people become scared, confused, or unsure of a situation. Signs of worry, nervousness, fidgeting, and/or paranoia are

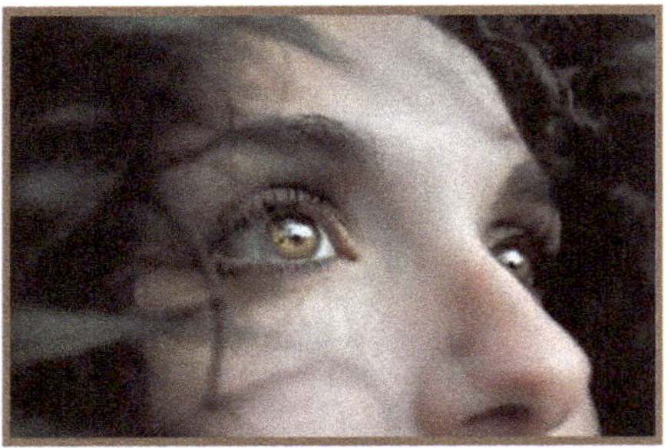

some noticeable behaviors. Those with dementia are simply trying to express their feelings when reason and words can no longer be used to communicate their needs.

When *fright* is a factor, a common behavior is for our loved ones to hide things. They are aware that their life isn't right; they know they are losing control and may be afraid they may lose their possessions. Don't bother asking why something is missing or where they put it; they will not remember hiding it or where it is. Instead, they will often blame someone else for stealing their belongings, such as a housekeeper or family member.

Caregiver response: ______________________…VALIDATE…REDIRECT.

Flight mode: When it becomes clear that a person wants to remove themselves from their current situation and environment, *flight is* their way of telling us that they are confused about where they are, unhappy, mentally lost, extremely uneasy, and/or uncomfortable. As they search for escape from their situation, their behaviors result in their wanting to leave the room, wanting to go home, or stubbornness and/or wandering.

Caregiver response: REWIND…_________________…REDIRECT.

It is imperative for caregivers to have a safety plan in place if their loved one tends to wander.

When your person continually asks to go home, they are expressing feelings of insecurity, anxiety, and depression. *Home* reflects long-term memories of times and places when they were calm and secure. Due to memory loss, nothing may feel familiar anymore and the person subconsciously is just connecting home with a sense of familiarity and belonging.

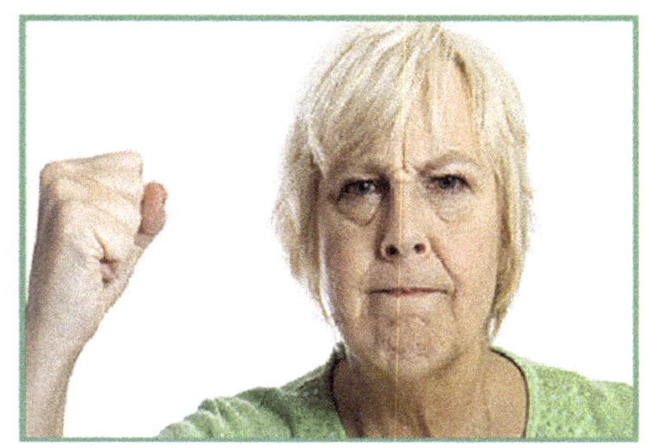

Fight mode: Loved ones are sometimes combative, agitated, unreasonable, or speaking in nasty tones that can escalate into yelling, swearing, making threats, etc. In reality, they are desperately expressing intense anger about something. This can be due to anything they find unfair, confusing, annoying, or threatening. It can also be medical in nature, so their anger can be triggered by things like constipation, aches, pains, or urinary tract infection (UTI).

Caregiver response: REWIND…VALIDATE…_________________.

Severe combative agitation can occur in the *fight* mode, and separation from emotional intensity may be needed. *Your loved one will not be the person you know and love.* Exhibited behaviors include physical aggression, verbal aggression, anxiety, paranoia, irritability, extreme frustration, and discomfort.

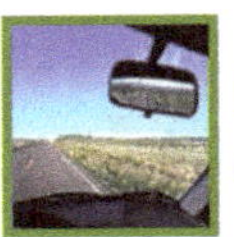

Expanding your horizons

Agitation 1: Behaviors

Read aloud *MTM BOOK*, page 59, first two paragraphs.
Review examples of agitated behaviors and triggers: *MTM BOOK*, pages 59–60.

- Agitation-caused behaviors

- Medical-caused behaviors

- Daily life-caused behaviors

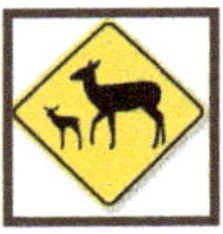

"Dears" Crossing: reflection and discussion

Agitation 1: behaviors

Which of these behaviors have you seen your loved one exhibit?

What behaviors did you exhibit in response?

The illness is creating the behavior, not the person you once knew. You will never be able to separate your emotional connection from your loved one's emotional behavior, but the suggested 5 R's of Dementia Care will help you from worsening the situation.

Agitation 2: Emotional Intensity

Read *MTM BOOK*, page 61.

The 5 R's of Dementia Care:

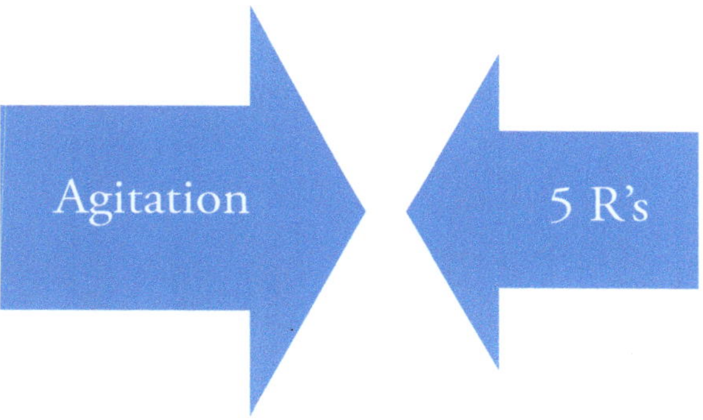

- **R**emain calm
- **R**espond to feelings
- **R**eassure
- **R**emove
- **R**eturn

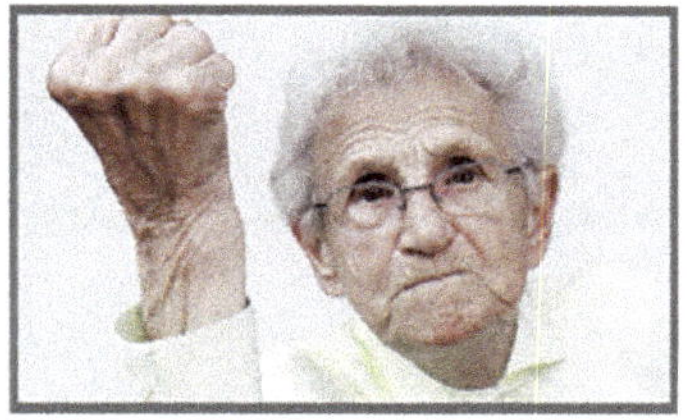

As those with cognitive impairment decline, agitation behaviors will occur. Some may be mild, and others may escalate and become extremely disruptive or even dangerous.

(Homewatch CareGivers)

When _____________________, situations occur. QUICKLY review the **5 R's of Dementia Care,** Appendix D.

Copy and keep in an accessible place to use when needed.

Read Aloud "The Cardiologist," an agitation story, ***MTM BOOK***, pages 68–69.

Agitation 2

What were the three levels of agitation that created overwhelming triggers for Brandon?

His responses are good examples of combative behaviors that could be calmed using the 5 R's approach.

Have you seen this type of agitation with your loved one?

How could using the 5 R's of Dementia Care be helpful to you when agitation situations occur in the future?

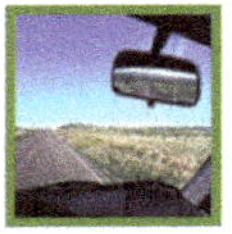 **Expanding your horizons**

Agitation 3: Sundowning

Sundown syndrome is a neurological phenomenon associated with increased confusion and restlessness in patients with some form of dementia and it is most common with Alzheimer's disease. Behavioral problems occur in the evening or while the sun is setting and it occurs more frequently during the middle stages of dementia.

Sundown syndrome is an area where validation and redirection are often used. A further study is necessary to clarify behaviors, triggers, and care approaches.

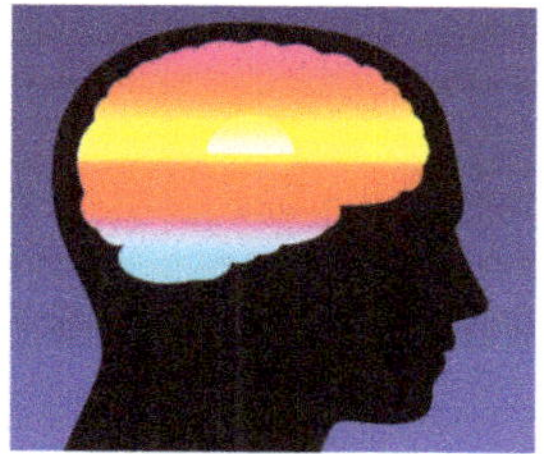

Sundowning seems to develop suddenly as evening approaches. Your loved one may be doing fine in the afternoon and then seem to become a different person as the sun sets. When community staff are asked about the personality of a patient, a day shift worker and an evening shift worker might describe the person totally differently. Thus, caregivers may need to use different approaches depending on the time of day. This disorder affects those with dementia and occasionally some people that have no cognitive impairment.

(Verywell Health)

Sundowning behaviors include restlessness, falls, pandering, wandering, calling out, crying, yelling, fearfulness, paranoia, mood swings, hallucinations, and shadowing.

Sundowning triggers include fatigue, boredom, loneliness, overstimulation, hunger, chronic pain, medication, fear of unknown people, seasonal lighting changes, unmet needs, caregiver stress, and burnout.

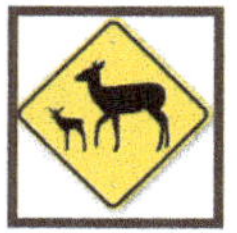 **"Dears" Crossing: reflection and discussion**

Agitation 3: sundowning

Have you noticed any sundowning behaviors in your loved one? How can validation and redirection skills be used when sundowning behaviors occur? Review these redirection techniques in the *JG*, page 46–49.

53

What situations in your journey do you think you might handle differently if you focused on making your ________________ ____________________ feel confirmed, verified, supported, and validated?

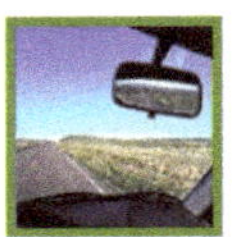

Expanding your horizons

Open Arms

Open arms is a positive action approach that allows ________________ to be a major factor in communication.

Debbie Selsavage, an expert in dementia, suggests that extending *OPEN ARMS* without touching or invading a person's space can build trust, love, and kindness.

This gesture is a key element in controlling *flight, freight,* and *fight* situations because it initiates general calmness. This nonverbal arm extension does not require hearing, speaking, or a cognitive challenge for those with dementia.

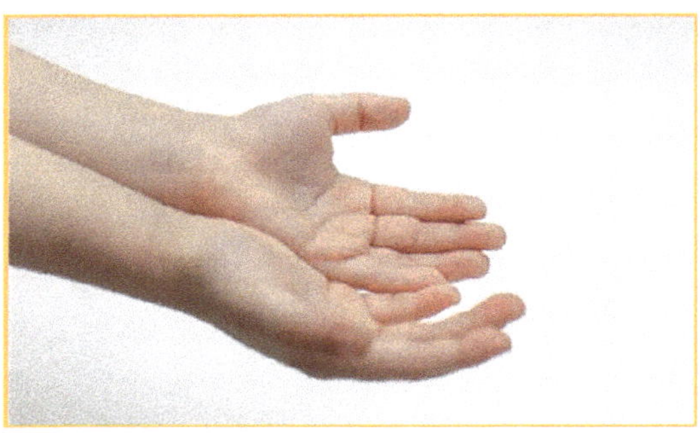

It is a great practice to begin using this approach during normal daily living situations, such as greetings, requests to go somewhere, or even giving affection.

Allow your loved one to reach out to you before touching them so a trust-based relationship can be established.

Feelings of threat or fear are a common response for those with cognitive decline whenever they do not recognize someone or when their space is invaded. Encourage and teach staff, family members, friends, and strangers to use the open-arm approach.

Turning to the Word of God

Jesus's arms are open wide for all to come. This image reminds us how LOVE can bring comfort, peace, and a trust-based relationship with God as well as to those on the caregiver journey.

> "Take my yoke upon you and learn from me, for I am gentle and humble in heart, and you will find rest for your souls." (Matthew 11:29 NIV)

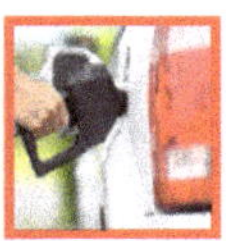

Care for the caregiver

Journaling

The University of Iowa's School of Nursing conducted a writing study. They found that journaling during stressful events promotes better health.

Journaling reduces stress and gives the immune system a boost. Outcomes from writing studies show that caregivers that journal made _______________________ trips to the doctor.

> **At-Home Study**
>
> Review *MTM BOOK*, page 19, "Moment Components."
> **For future meeting**, read *MTM BOOK*, pages 73–75.

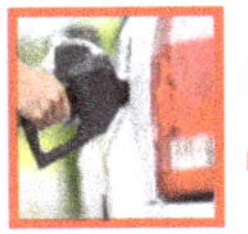 **Care for the caregiver**

Journaling 2: The Notebook

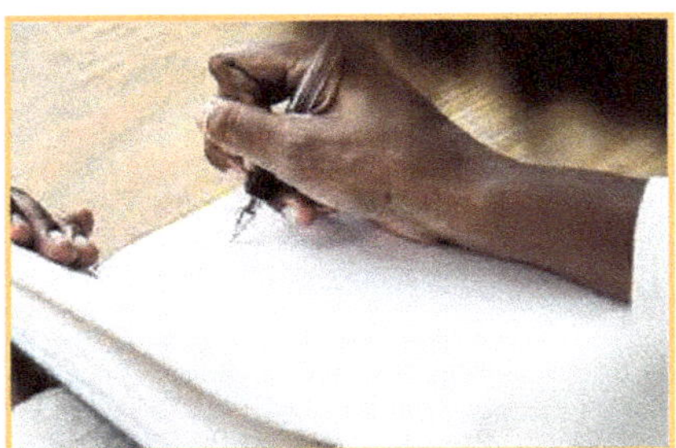

Clearly, caregiving keeps us extremely busy and often exhausted by day's end, but it is worth the effort to find time to record parts of your journey.

Keep a small notebook to jot down quick specifics about your loved one. Record things such as weight loss or gain, eating habits, physical mobility, prescription changes, declining cognitive skills, abilities, loss of interest in activities, and behavioral changes. This is a good way to clarify changes for yourself, doctors, or family members.

It is crucial for caregivers to remain healthy. Personal journaling is another way of caring for our mental health by releasing the negative feelings of being overwhelmed, frustrated, guilty, or angry. This is important since carrying the baggage of negative emotions can lead to depression, anxiety, and fear.

So make time and take time to express your thoughts, emotions, and behaviors by writing them down. At day's end, remove all your bad feelings and release your frustrations on paper. Always empty your emotional bottle before going to bed.

Whatever you are feeling is perfectly normal on this long and bumpy caregiver journey. Remember, we are the boat people, all in the same boat, and these negative emotions are inevitable and valid, and there is no room for self-blame or guilt.

When you and your pen are done venting, take a nice deep breath, and slowly reread what you have written. Try to look objectively at what you have expressed, and consider ways to convert your negative energy into opportunities for change and growth if the same situation should present itself again.

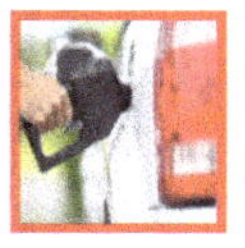 **Care for the caregiver**

Journaling 3: Mount your Fishes!

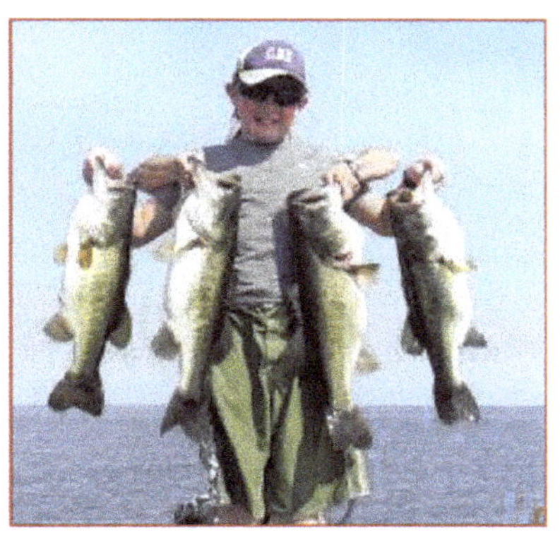

We have already discussed the first two types of journaling, the loved one's notebook and the caregiver's personal journal. The third type is one I call *Mount your Fishes!*

Did you ever know someone that had a trophy room? It probably was filled with the head of a deer or an elk with a large impressive rack. It might have had a beautiful, stuffed pheasant or even a small shark. Sports trophies, diplomas, and blue ribbons might have been proudly hung on the wall, or they might be lined with celebratory photographs of life's best moments, weddings, graduations, and family gatherings. All these things big or small represent a moment when people were basking in the sun with pride and glory. These are things deemed worthy of remembering or sharing.

Mount your fishes! Start with a journal-type calendar, and record something positive that God blessed you with the day before. Any tiny triumph, a word of affirmation, or a whispered "I love you" might be a really big fish in your trophy room. A breakthrough, an enjoyed activity, a successful outing, a few minutes of peace instead of frustration, or someone appreciating all you do should be noted. Some days, my recorded *fish* was getting a good parking space at the doctor's office or spying a new bloom in my garden. At the end of each month, I have a calendar that is full of God's blessings, none of which were too small to record. Be ready to give God glory, and encourage others as you share your trophy room of joy.

Caregiver JOY journaling is beneficial in several ways. It allows you to look back and recall happy moments at any given time. This is especially important on your most challenging days. Reading these heartfelt words will remind you of the good work you are doing and that there really is a positive side to caregiving. It will lift your spirits, give you hope, and encourage you to move forward.

It allows you to appreciate the ________________________ in your loved one.

It will give you a ________________________ to share with family and friends. Allow them to visit your trophy room by sharing positive stories. These will create nice memories for everyone.

It will help you to encourage and support other ________________________.

After expressing your emotions in your journal, take the next step, and give it to God. Our caregiver scripture verse, *JG*, page 3, is as follows:

"Come to me all you are weary and burdened, and I will give you rest." (Matthew 11:28 NIV)

This is a promise verse. When you come to him, he will give you rest. If you do your part, Jesus promises to do his. Keep it by your bedside. And read it, and pray it each night. Let Jesus give you rest after a long day and strength for the new day to come. It will be helpful to memorize this verse. It will bring comfort when you are feeling burdened.

Take a look back

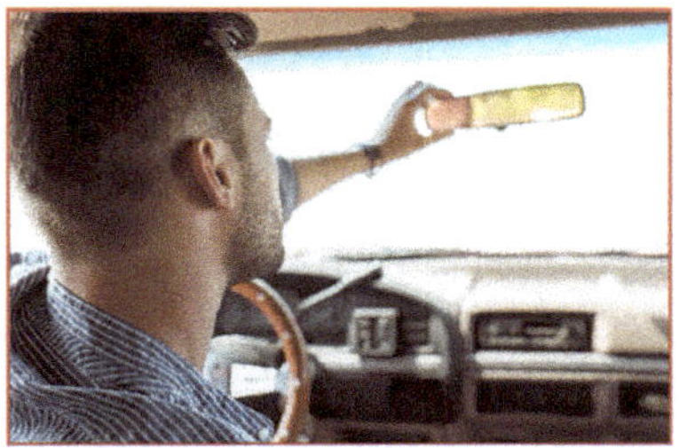

Read the *Moment-Method*: "Moment Components," *MTM BOOK*, page 19.

The *Moment-Method* includes three components that are needed to make successful *Moments that Matter*. If one of these three is missing, the moment will fail to be significant.

Components 1 and 2: Changes and Stages

Observation of your loved ones' changes and stages is extremely important.

Caregivers must accept their person's changes and then adapt and change themselves. It is imperative for the caregiver to become aware and familiar with the stages and symptoms of physical and cognitive decline.

Successful moments enhance the quality of life of our loved ones.

The three components needed to create *Moments that Matter* are ___________________, ___________________, and an enjoyed activity.

Component 3: Enjoyed Activities

Activities are not meant to provide busyness; they are meant to be enjoyed. **Read aloud** *MTM BOOK*, page 73, the last paragraph.

Moments that Matter are the creation of short meaningful connections between a caregiver and their loved one.

These connections bring JOY to both the loved ones and the caregivers!

 **"Dears" Crossing: reflection and discussion**

Enjoyed activities

Read aloud the story, "Activities Outside The Box," *MTM BOOK*, page 74.

What parts of this story's *moments* were beneficial to the loved one's well-being?

Brainstorm and discuss some other activities that might provide sensory involvement, purpose, self-esteem building, stress-free cognitive challenges, reminiscing, and engagement.

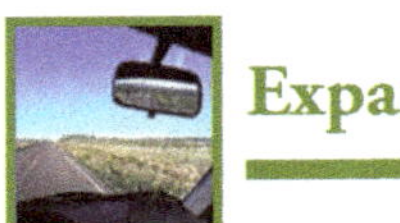

Expanding your horizons

Enjoyed Activities

Read aloud and consider the activity categories listed in *MTM BOOK*, page 75. Begin to think about what your loved one might enjoy. Each category provides many activity ideas and options. Clearly, our loved ones are all unique. Therefore, everyone will not enjoy all activities. However, all the activity suggestions in *MTM BOOK* can be adapted so that all moments will be _____________________ and _____________________ appropriate.

I have found that the following activity categories are enjoyed by most people:

- Reminisce: *MTM BOOK*, pages 98–99.

This is a way to focus on your loved one's past. If you recall, long-term memories are remembered much longer than short-term ones. All the suggestions are engaging. Start conversations using the words "tell me" or "show me" so those with memory loss can share whatever they remember rather than having to answer probing questions that ask who, what, why, when, or where. All the activities can be adapted for individual needs, and many of them can be used again to create successful memories.

- Games and puzzles: *MTM BOOK*, pages 108–112

There are games and puzzles for all ages and abilities. Choose ones that you and your loved one can enjoy together.

- Laughter: *MTM BOOK*, pages 113–114

Get your clown nose out!

> Laughter is seen with the eyes, heard with the ears and felt with the heart. When you open the mind to laugh, you open the mind to learn. (Boltz)

- Spirit and cheer it: *MTM BOOK*, pages 117–125

Spirituality, purpose, and self-image are the three parts of this category. These are all very important for maintaining a good quality of life for those with cognitive decline. Study these suggestions carefully and intentionally incorporate them when creating *Moments that Matter*.

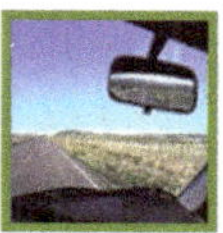

Expanding your horizons

Enjoyed Activities: Exercise

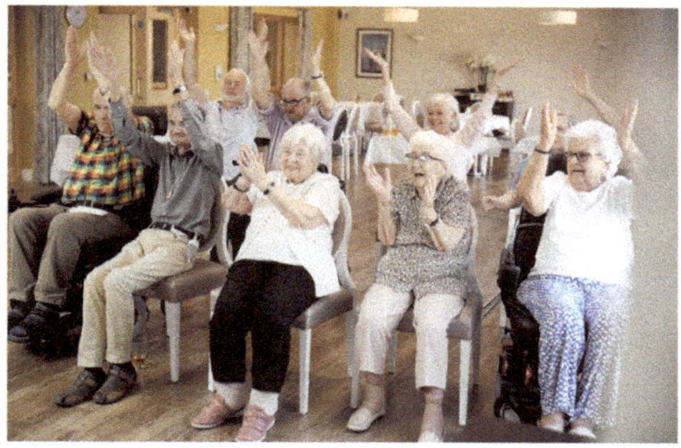

Read "General Exercise," *MTM BOOK*, pages 101–103.

A complete head-to-toe exercise routine is in *MTM BOOK*, pages 101–102.

Routine exercise helps to maintain the body and the hippocampus, the part of the brain that controls memory. All exercise must be done _____________________ and appropriately for each individual.

This is a seated program that can be done in any chair and is easy to adapt according to your person's abilities. Doing these together a few times a week is an easy way to establish an ongoing *Moments that Matter* activity.

Consult your doctor and carefully determine how strenuous the workout should be before beginning. A gradual progression is usually recommended.

The health benefits of exercise for caregivers and their loved ones are as follows:

- Improved cognitive impairment: Any physical activity, including walking, that requires attention, coordination, and/or navigational skills can improve selective functions in most older adults.

- Lessening depression symptoms: Physical exercise immolates the production of hormones and neurotransmitters associated with memory and mood. It can help elevate moods and enhance memory training.

- Improved balance: _____________________ and fractures affect those with Alzheimer's three times more than other people.

- Prevention of cardiovascular complications: Routine exercise, along with diet, weight loss, and the cessation of smoking, is central to the prevention and treatment of cardiovascular diseases associated with diminished blood flow to the brain.

- Improved sleep patterns: Even in perfectly healthy people, sleep deprivation is associated with fatigue, irritability, depression, lack of motivation, clumsiness, forgetfulness, and difficulty learning new concepts. Exercising with moderate intensity during the day makes it more likely that you will sleep at night. This may alleviate some lack of focus and confusion for those with memory loss. (Esther Heerema)

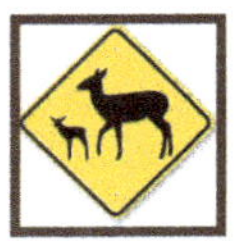 **"Dears" Crossing: reflection and discussion**

How many or all of these six exercise benefits might improve the life of your person?

How many or all of these six exercise benefits might improve your life?

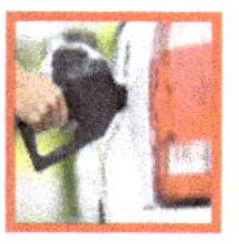

Care for the caregiver

Exercise

As Nike says, "Just do it!" A fun-and-easy way to get started is for support group members to become accountability partners. Check on each other or exercise on zoom.

As you begin an exercise program with your loved one, be sure to laugh and enjoy each other as you create meaningful quality time. The benefits are win-win! As the exercise routine is mastered, there are fun ways to add music and props. Read *MTM BOOK*, pages 102–103.

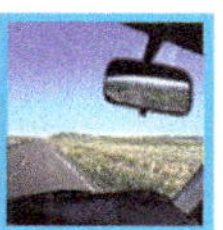

Expanding your horizons

Enjoyed activities 4: music

Read aloud "Karaoke Jay," *MTM BOOK*, page 124.

Musical moments gave a troubled man a meaningful purpose. He lifted spirits and unlocked the minds of those with cognitive decline.

Music can be used in many ways. I suggest getting creative by tapping into your person's long-term memories. Determine the specific music that was enjoyed during their lifetime. Whether it is old hymns, dance music, rock, opera, country songs, nursery rhymes, lullabies, or camp and childhood songs, music has the ability to bring enjoyment, joy, and quality to life.

Read music, *MTM BOOK*, pages 102–106.

There are many additional musical ideas within these pages. This activity category is one that can easily include others and is especially rewarding when it becomes an intergenerational activity.

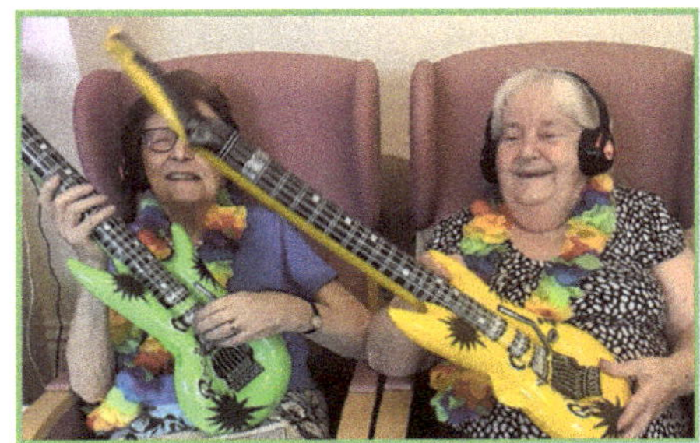

> "Music is used with elderly persons to increase or maintain their level of physical, mental and socio/emotional functioning. The sensory and intellectual stimulation of music is a person's quality of life." (Susan Warchol)

During the fifteen years I worked as a senior health-care activities director, I found music to be a miracle key that reached people with memory loss.

Read aloud "The Miracle Key," *MTM BOOK*, page 123.

> "Music has the ability to enhance people's brain connections with memories. People with Alzheimer's disease and other dementias can respond to music when nothing else reaches them. These illnesses can destroy the ability to remember family members or events from one's own life. Musical memory somehow survives the ravages of the disease and can even reach people with advanced dementia. Music can often ___________________ personal memories and associations otherwise lost." (Oliver Sacks).

"Sing to the Lord with grateful praise; make music to our God on the harp." (Psalm 147:7 NIV)

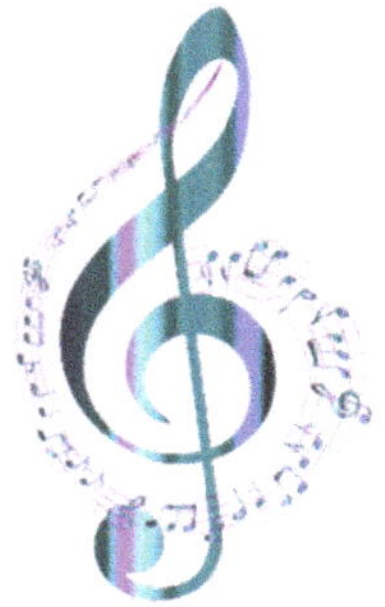

As spiritual people, we have been given the ability to express praise and worship to the Lord with songs and musical instruments.

As caregivers, let us travel on our challenging journey singing and listening to songs of worship and praise that will _______________ our souls in times of joy and sorrow.

 **"Dears" Crossing: reflection and discussion**

We learned that the *MTM BOOK* includes many activity choices that are likely to make successful *Moments that Matter* for most people.

To review, they are reminiscing, games and puzzles, laughter, spirituality, purpose, self-image, exercise, and music.

Which of these categories might be a good next step for you to create moments with your person? Share your ideas together.

When making moments, intentionally incorporate these activity categories and any others of interest to you and your loved one.

Take a look ahead. Create moments of joy for you and your loved one!

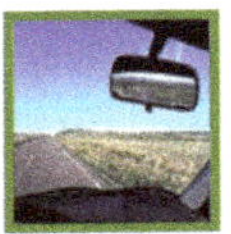

Expanding your horizons

Late-Stage Activities

Review the Dementia Stages Chart, *MTM BOOK*, pages 14-15.

When the symptoms of moderate and severe dementia become apparent in your loved one's life, moment-making will become more challenging for the caregiver.

No caregiver wants to imagine or experience that horrible day when their loved one doesn't know them. Every dementia journey is different, but the following suggestions may prolong memory retention and family facial recognition.

Send labeled photographs often and especially in advance of visits. Loading old and new photos to a digital frame are just an email away. Place this frame in your person's home where it can be continuously seen. When you or others are there, share a running commentary of people and events in the photos. I used this technique with my mother for seven years, and because of the constant repetition, she was able to remember her parents and cousins very well. And we were blessed that she recognized my sisters and me as she approached 102 years old.

During the length of your visit, crazy as it may seem, wear a large name and relationship tag around your neck. Always present an introduction, smile, compliment, and hug when you enter and leave the house.

Sometimes conversations may seem awkward or impossible during visits. Storytelling is an excellent way to trigger memories. Try verbally sharing your loved one's life story, singing songs or reading children's books and Bible stories. They will hear you, and it's very possible they will remember your voice. There might not always be verbal interaction; but nods, smiles, and a hand-squeeze can provide treasured communication. These times can be *moments that matter* to caregivers and their loved ones.

If there are times when your loved one does not know your name, it can still be an emotionally valued moment for you just to be perceived as someone they like and are happy to see.

Never try to correct what and who your loved ones may or may not know. Caregivers, it will be difficult, but enjoy and love them in whatever stage of life they are living in. And lastly, never give up. There may be lucid days when they know exactly who you are.

Hospice

It is wise to take advantage of hospice during the severe stages of dementia. *Hospice* is a word that is often misunderstood. It simply means making a unique care plan for your loved one. Physical, emotional, spiritual, and financial needs are provided by a team of doctors, nurses, companions, pastors, social workers, and volunteers. They also provide supplies and equipment, and most costs are covered by Medicare and Medicaid. Hospice care can be arranged in-home, in-facility, in a hospice house, or in a hospital. The main goal of hospice care is to provide comfort when your loved one's life expectancy is measured in months, not years.

I would like to express my gratitude to my mother's hospice nurse, Joanne Pennington. She provided skill, compassion, laughter, and excellence during every step of my mother's late-stage medical journey. Mom was unresponsive for the last few days of her life, but I knew in my heart she waited to breathe her last breath until she was on duty.

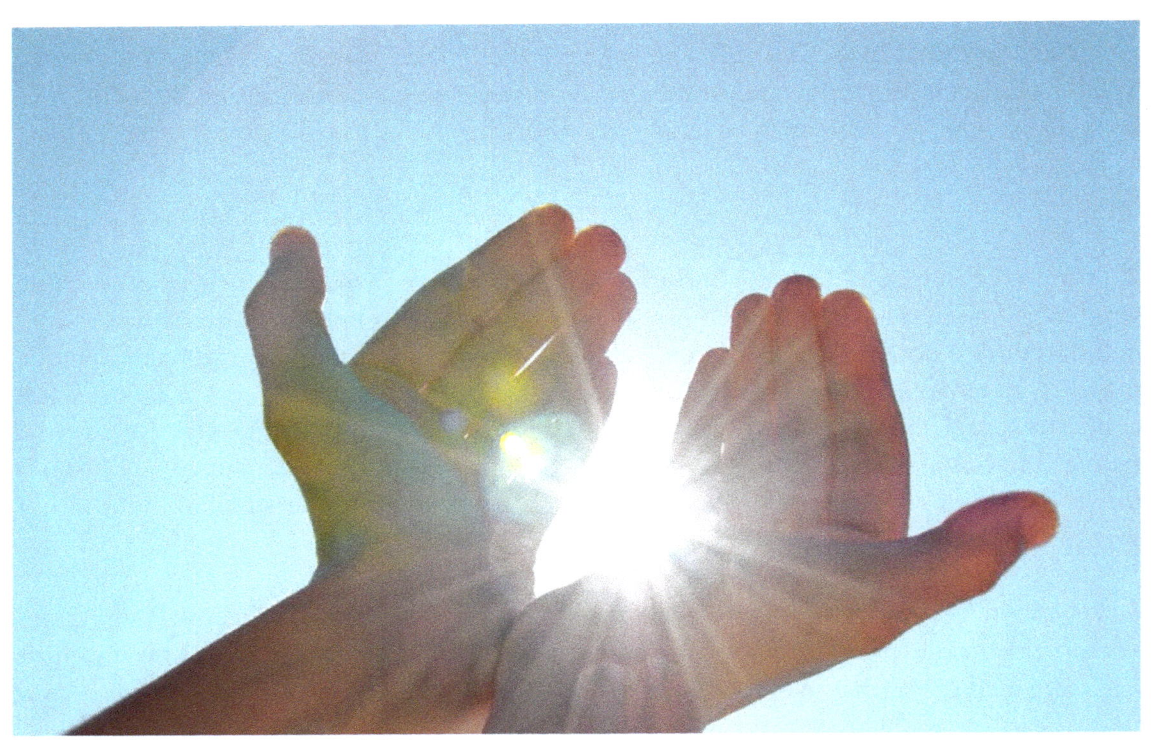

"*Life is not measured by the number of breaths we take...*

but by the moments that take our breath away."
—Maya Angelou

Appendix

Journey Guide Answer Key

Page 3
worship
blessed

Page 4
slowly
decline

Page 6
learn
denial
acceptance
themselves

Page 13
awareness
meaningful
connections

Page 14
three

Page 15
engaged
three

Page 16
components

Page 18
cognitive
advance
planning

Page 19
memory
retention

Page 22
unchecked

Page 27
cannot

Page 28
self-esteem
upsets

Page 29
laughter

Page 31
angry

Page 32
sight

Page 33
imbalance
same

Page 34
changes

Page 35
cognitive
abilities

Page 36
communication
reason
frustration

Page 38
advance

Page 40
negative

Page 42
pray

Page 43
listen

Page 44
feelings

Page 45
support
system
worship

Page 47
redirection

Page 48
trigger
Fright
Flight
Fight
Rewind

Page 49
Validate
Redirect

Page 51
combative

Page 54
loved
one
love

Page 55
fewer

Page 58
beauty
testimony
caregivers

Page 60
changes
stages

Page 62
age
ability

Page 63
safely

Page 64
falls

Page 66
revive

Page 67
fuel

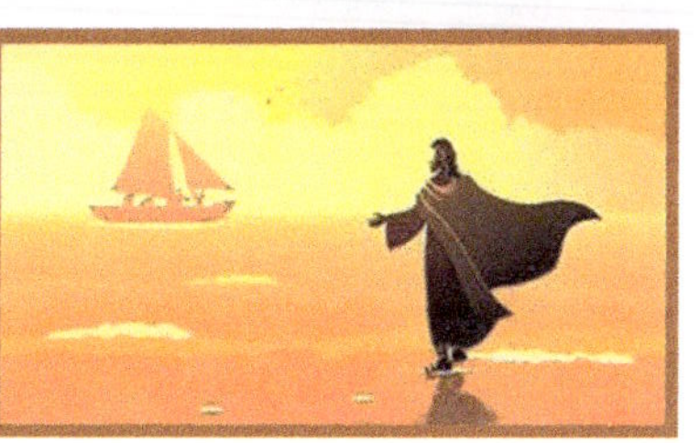

Boat Card

Hang this *affirmation card* where you can see it often—on the mirror, dashboard, kitchen cabinet, etc.

Each time you read it, you will be reminded that *you are not alone.*

Seek God during hard times, and *praise him* on both good and bad days.

Caregiver Scripture Verse: a nightly reminder of God's promise.

Scripture Verse

(Matthew 11:28 NIV)

"Come to me all you are weary and burdened, and I will give you rest."

Scripture Bookmark

(Matthew 8:23–27 NIV) *Jesus Calms the Storm*

"Then he got into the boat and his disciples followed him. Without warning, a furious storm came up on the lake, so the waves went over the boat. But Jesus was sleeping. The disciples went and woke him saying, "Lord we are going to drown!" He replied, "You of little faith, why are you so afraid?" Then he got up and rebuked the wind and the waves, and it was completely calm. The men were amazed and asked, "What kind of man is this? Even the wind and waves obey him."

We learn in this passage that we, as caregivers, can have peace knowing that when "caregiver storms" arise with fury, anger, and frustrations, **we can go to Jesus**. Even the wind and the waves obey him, and **He will calm our storms**. He will save us from drowning—Jesus is in our boat. **(We are not alone, we are the "Boat People," supporting each other, with God's power and love as our center.).**

Moments that Matter: **Holiday Tips**

Enhance the quality of your loved ones' life during seasonal gatherings.

- **Connect:** Encourage family members, in advance, to include compliments and affection when greeting your loved one. Do not let them sit on the sidelines and have celebrations around them.
- **Purpose:** "The purpose of life is not to be happy. It is to be useful, honorable, to have it make a difference that you have lived and lived well" (Ralph Waldo Emerson).
- Regardless if you need help, find a task for your loved one. Give them a purpose! Always use "self-esteem"-building words, such as "I need your help," "Will you help me?" "I couldn't have done this without you," or "You are the best helper ever!"

Holiday Purpose Suggestions

- **In the kitchen:** Can your loved one stir the batter, break the eggs, use cookie cutters, or sprinkle sugar? Can they help color eggs at Easter?
- **Holiday helpers:** Can they wrap small items, cut the paper, stick-on tags, cross things off lists, or hold their finger for you to knot a ribbon? Can your loved one put grass and candy in baskets or help hide eggs for a family Easter egg hunt? If they need to just sit in an easy chair, have them hold a big basket, and the children can bring them all the eggs they find.
- **Decorating:** Can loved ones help decorate the tree, unwrap ornaments, or put them on hooks? Can they help set the holiday tables?
- **Engage:** How can everyone be included? Create activities that are age and ability appropriate. Intergenerational events are great. Children are especially loved by older family members and often bring special joy to special occasions.

Holiday Engagement Suggestions

- Watch holiday movies, especially ones with singing and dancing. Make popcorn, and hold hands. Lavish love, and cheer on loved ones.
- Take a drive, and see holiday decorations in the community. Sing songs, and reminisce with photographs and stories. Pray together, and read stories.
- Other ideas for holiday fun and family gatherings can be found in *MTM BOOK*, pages 115–116 and on pages 24–25.

The 5 R's of Dementia Care:

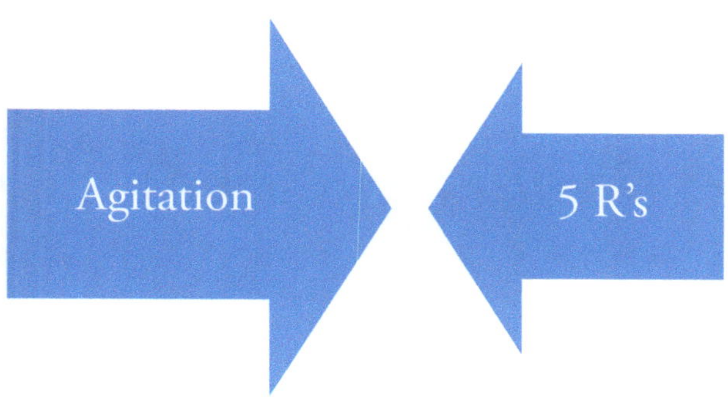

- **R**emain calm
- **R**espond to feelings
- **R**eassure
- **R**emove
- **R**eturn

As those with cognitive impairment decline, agitation behaviors will occur. Some may be mild, and others may escalate and become extremely disruptive or even dangerous. (Homewatch CareGivers)

When combative situations occur, QUICKLY review the **5 R's of Dementia Care**.

Copy and keep this in an accessible place to use when needed.

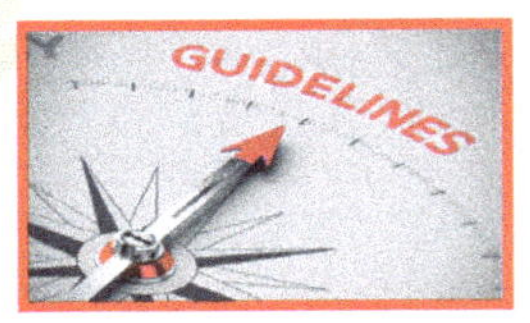

Moments that Matter

Caregiver Support Group Guidelines

Engage:

Confidentiality

Memory loss support groups must be particularly sensitive in the area of confidentiality. General dementia and caregiver learning opportunities can be shared with others. However, any specifics about individual group members must stay within the group.

Member issues easily lead to medical conversations and discussions, so awareness of HIPAA laws should be observed. If members choose to share some specific information, they are giving group members permission to receive this medical information.

Sharing

It is a great benefit to each group member to share the successes and challenges of their journey with other people who understand, care, and are in the *same boat*.

Sensitivity

Because we all have different personalities, there will always be different dynamics in each group. If, for example, you are more reserved, please make every effort to share and participate. If, on the other hand, you are more outgoing, please try not to dominate discussions.

Everyone has valuable insights to share. It is the facilitator's job to give each person the opportunity to speak during every session. This is how support groups build solid, caring relationships.

During group discussions, the facilitator may need to redirect an outgoing speaker that begins to monopolize the conversation. They may subtly say, "Thanks for you your input, Mary" and *quickly say to another member*, "Jane, do you have anything to add to that?" or "John, we haven't heard from you today."

Communication between meetings

Do pray for the group on a regular basis, and encourage each other when possible. Send prayer requests and praise reports, via email or text, to the facilitator or members.
The facilitator will be open to giving a needed resource, a word of encouragement, or prayer as a response to a member's email or quick phone call. However, *a support group is not meant to include private counseling.*

Goal

To provide needed support and spiritual encouragement to one another as we travel our caregiver journeys together.

Member Information Form

Name _________________________ Phone _________________________ Email Address _________________________

This is all about you. Check which statement best describes your interest in this group.

1. _______ I am a caregiver for a loved one. Who is your loved one?

   Circle all that apply.

   My loved one is my spouse, my parent, other family member, my friend, my neighbor, or other _______________.

2. My loved one:
   _______ lives with me
   _______ lives in their own home
   _______ lives in an assisted living, memory care or other community

3. I am with my loved one: _______ full time. _______ part time

4. _______ In addition to being a caregiver, I have a job.
   _______ full time
   _______ part time

5. I am a paid professional caregiver:
   _______ private duty
   _______ in a community

6. I am involved with seniors in another way. How? _________________________

7. _______ I am not a caregiver, but I have an interest in learning about memory loss.

8. _______ Other _________________________

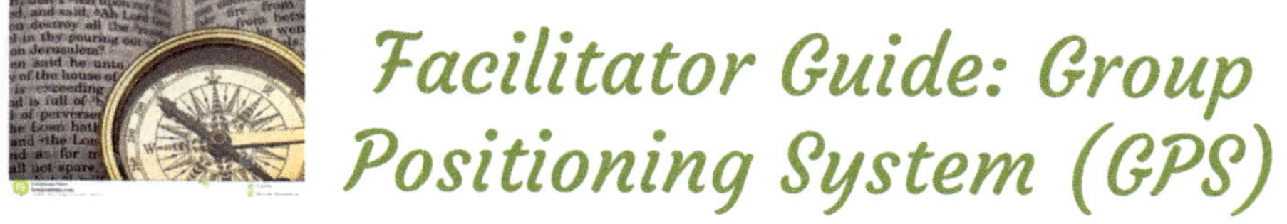

Facilitator Guide: Group Positioning System (GPS)

Facilitator Support

Caregiver group leaders are always welcome to contact Karen Cochran Beaulieu with any questions, suggestions, or concerns about their group at www.moment-making.com or momentsthatmatterkcb@gmail.com

Group Venue

Due to COVID-19, there are two choices, Zoom Meetings or In-Person Meetings.

Zoom Meetings are preferred by many caregivers and leaders because:

- loved ones are usually high risk so health protection is important and necessary,

- strong group relationships are established,

- no need to arrange for someone to stay with loved ones while away at a meeting,

- no travel time or gas usage, and

- no need to dress up, so come as you are!

There is a $14.99 monthly fee for Zoom leader ownership that allows unlimited time periods for meetings. Most churches should have this type of Zoom available. If not, the cost is easily offset since there is no travel and setup time required.

In-Person Meetings are preferred by many facilitators and caregivers because face-to-face interaction is a more personal way to establish relationships.

Some group members are more comfortable in this situation. However, be aware that in-person meetings will be a mixed group, and every member will have made medical choices about vaccinations.

Member Venue Feedback

A short phone or email conversation in advance will allow the facilitator to attain preferences for a venue and meeting times and gain information about the member's caregiver situation.

Choose Time Frames

A definite day of week and time should be established for every other week meetings. The session time is one and a half hours.

- For example, on the second and fourth Thursdays of each month, 5:30–7:00 p.m. This time slot allows working caregivers to come after work.

- Gives members a choice to eat supper before or after the meeting.

- The meeting will not last until late into the evening, which might interfere with the bedtime habits of loved ones.

Facilitator Follow-Up Communication by Phone

- Share venue decisions and meeting times.

- During this phone conversation, facilitators should complete the **member information form,** Appendix F, with each person that makes a commitment to join the group. Five minutes past the start time, the facilitator will begin **group member introductions** by using each person's individual information that was gathered during their advance communication.

- How to use these member information forms at a meeting is explained under the heading *Introductions* below.

Introductions

Since allowing group members to introduce themselves can often get lengthy and off track, the leader will present each member as shown by using the examples below. Note how varied a group can be and why sharing each person's individual situation is so valuable to form relationships:

- I'm Karen, your group facilitator. I worked in senior health care for fifteen years and have been a family caregiver for both my mother and father-in-law.

- This is April. She is a caregiver for her husband in their home on a 24-7 basis.

- This is Marie. She is a caregiver for her mother who lives in an assisted living.

- This is Jason. He works full time and is a family caregiver for his father, who lives in another state. His contacts are made by phone calls, Zoom visits, and occasional in-person visits, mostly on holidays.

- This is Bryan. He is a part-time caregiver for his neighbor.

Members will begin to get acquainted quickly and relationships will grow.

Required texts

Facilitators should email these titles to each group member, and books should be purchased before the first meeting:

- *Moments that Matter; a roadmap for caregivers and their loved ones with memory loss* (*MTM*)
- *Moments that Matter: A Companion Journey Guide for Caregiver Support Groups or Individual Study* (*JG*)

Books can be previewed and purchased at Amazon Books and wherever books are sold. Search: Cochran Beaulieu

A video text introduction is available on YouTube. Search: Cochran Beaulieu.

Meeting structure

This group's framework has been deliberately designed to be "ongoing." I have found that within the hearts of caregivers dwells such an *interest* and *hunger* to seek ways to make their caregiver journeys easier and more meaningful and that hurried agendas, individual lessons, or class time parameters aren't necessary.

Therefore, lessons and meetings are continuous and have no specific beginning or end, but rather, the group can flow at the pace of its members. Some topics may prompt more emotional feelings and conversation than others. Sometimes, "smaller bites" will be necessary for complete "digestion" and understanding of any given information. Sometimes, member support needs will be intense, and it will take more time for meaningful discussion.

The **ninety-minute** start-and-finish time should be strictly adhered to, but there should never be pressure to quickly gloss over or to even skip part of the text. Be assured that complete sharing, learning, and support will continue "right where you left off" at the next meeting.

The Word of God is woven throughout the journey pathway. Scriptures provide comfort, encouragement, suggestions, and self-care for caregivers.

For the first meeting, follow the *Journey Guide*, page 9.

Welcome

As people arrive, facilitators should give a general welcome and identify themselves:

- In-person: Give them a name tag, and double-check that their information form is correct.

- On Zoom: Names will automatically appear on screens.

Guidelines

- Review the group guidelines together in Appendix E, pages 76–77.

- Emphasize the sections on confidentiality, listening, and group sensitivity.

- Facilitators should give each person the opportunity to share if they wish during every session. This is an important part of a good support group.

- During group discussions, the facilitator may need to redirect a speaker that begins to monopolize the conversation. Kindly say, "Thanks for you your input, Mary," and *quickly say to another member*, "Jane, do you have anything to add to that?" or "John, we haven't heard from you today."

Communication between meetings

The facilitator should be open to responding to a member's email or quick phone call between meetings to give a resource, a word of encouragement, or prayer. However, remind members that a support group is not meant to include private counseling.

Review support group benefits in the table in *JG*, page 1.

Introduce *boat cards*: Have members detach the *boat card* page from the appendix, page, Appendix B. It will yield three separate cards as shown.

Affirmation Card

Scripture Bookmark: **Matthew 8:23–27 (NIV)**
Caregiver Scripture Verse: **Matthew 8:28 (NIV)**

We are the boat people!

Review each boat card individually with the group.

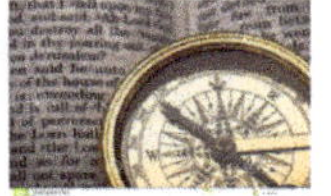 **Review** *How to Navigate the Journey Guide*, page xiii.

Explain how each road sign will be used throughout the *Journey Guide*. The first road sign, Turning to the Word of God, is on page 3 of the *Journey Guide*.

 **Turning to the Word of God**

"Come to me, all you who are weary and burdened, and I will give you rest." (Matthew 11:28 NIV)

Follow the *Journey Guide* on page 3 to unpack this verse and explain how it is to be used daily. **Introduce** the *Moments that Matter* text, pages 4.

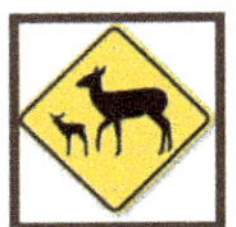 **"Dears" Crossing: reflection and discussion**

At this point, ask the group if anyone would like to share their biggest success or challenge during the past week. The facilitator should share first.

Let the discussion travel on its own. Group members will begin to ask questions, share, and discuss different feelings and problems.

> **At-Home Study**
>
> Assignments should be given in advance, so group members will be prepared for a future meeting, regardless of where you choose to end the meeting.
> **Prayer:** Allow time for spiritual support when choosing where to stop the discussion, and always end the meeting with prayer requests.
> *You are on the way* and now ready to proceed using the *MTM BOOK* and the *Journey Guide* together for future meetings.

Facilitator support

Caregiver group leaders are always welcome to contact Karen Cochran Beaulieu with any questions, suggestions, or concerns about their group at www.moment-making.com or momentsthatmatterkcb@gmail.com.

Bibliography

Alzheimer's Association. National Office, Chicago, Illinois. www.alz.org.

Alzheimer's Family Organization. Springhill, Florida. info@alzheimersfamily.org.

Boltz, Elaine. Certified laughter leader and wellness trainer. Lancaster area, PA.

Bains, Gurinder Singh. "The Effect of Humor on Short-Term Memory in Older: a New Component for Whole-Person Wellness." *Adv. Mind Body Med.* (2014).

Bible, Life Application Study NIV. Tyndale House

DBT Self Help. "Invalidation." www.dbtselfhelp.com.

Department of Health. Alzheimer's Victoria, Australia. "Dementia-Friendly Environments."

Heerema, Esther, MSW. "6 Ways That Exercise Helps Alzheimer's Disease." Very Well Health. February 2020.

Maya, Angelou. American poet, memoirist, and civil rights advocate.

Sacks, Oliver, CBE FRCP. British/American neurologist.

Sauer, Paul. "The 5 R's of Dementia Care." www. Homewatchcaregivers.org. 2014 web.

Selsavage, Debbie. Coping With Dementia LLC. www.deb@coping.today.

Scott, Paula Spencer. "18 Ways to Prolong Independence." www.caring.com.

Studer, Joanne Pitera, PSYD. Clinical psychologist. drjo@actions4life.com.

Verywell Health. www.verywellhealth.com.

Warchol, Susan, MFA. "Music Therapy." Goodwin College at Drexel University, Philadelphia, PA.

Willkomm, Anne Converse. MFA. "Communication skills." Goodwin College at Drexel University, Philadelphia, PA.